HOLLY healthiest diets

Protein Plus
40-40-20
Hi Low
1day Quick Fix

HOLLYWOOD'S
healthiest
diets

healthy fat-fighting diets

Dr. Tony Perrone
with Mark Laska

ReganBooks
An Imprint of HarperCollins*Publishers*

A hardcover edition of this book was published by ReganBooks in 1999 under the title *Dr. Tony Perrone's Body-Fat Breakthru.*

HOLLYWOOD'S HEALTHIEST DIETS. Copyright © 1999 by Dr. Tony Perrone. All rights reserved. Printed in the United States of America. No part of this book may be used or reproduced in any manner whatsoever without written permission except in the case of brief quotations embodied in critical articles and reviews. For information address HarperCollins Publishers Inc., 10 East 53rd Street, New York, NY 10022.

HarperCollins books may be purchased for educational, business, or sales promotional use. For information please write: Special Markets Department, HarperCollins Publishers Inc., 10 East 53rd Street, New York, NY 10022.

First ReganBooks/Perennial edition published 2000.

Designed by Interrobang Design Studio

The Library of Congress Cataloging-in-Publication Data for the hardcover edition is on file with the Library of Congress.

ISBN 0-06-039274-6

ISBN 0-06-098848-7 (pbk.)

00 01 02 03 04 ❖/RRD 10 9 8 7 6 5 4 3 2 1

This work is dedicated to my daughter,
Terra Marie Perrone,

CONTENTS

Recipes

ACKNOWLEDGMENTS

First and foremost I would like to thank God. He has blessed me with a very special gift, one that has allowed me to save lives, to enrich lives, to improve the quality of life for so many. God has also blessed me with a wonderful family, good friends, and a great life.

I must express my deepest, most heartfelt thanks to my mother Bonnie. She was a single mother who at times worked three jobs so that our family would never go without. She played the roles of Mom, Dad, Nanny, Housekeeper, Friend, Confidant, and so on. My mother did a fantastic job of raising us and I see her in my personality on a daily basis—which pleases me. I definitely would not be enjoying the wonderful life I have today if she did not so carefully tend to our family.

You would not be reading this book if not for the monumental efforts of my good friend, partner, and co-author, Mark Laska. He has sacrificed much to see this project through in a timely manner. Without Mark, I may have never finished this project. Mark's efforts have been continuous and significant for two years now, and I very much appreciate all he has done for me.

I am sincerely grateful to the many people who have entrusted me with their health and wellness over the past eight years. The experience I have gained through each case has made it possible for the next case to enjoy even greater benefit. Without them, this book could not have been written.

SPECIAL THANKS

Thanks to Keith Cubba for helping my practice to grow. Thanks to Kevin Lewis for believing in my abilities early on. Thanks to Lisa Ridino for managing my office so very efficiently and being dedicated to her work. Thanks to Dr. Vicki Sutherland for giving me a place to expand my abilities and the confidence she showed by referring her patients to me. Thanks to Mike and Sherri Ditto for all their support, even during some rough waters, and for giving me their daughter's hand in marriage. Thanks to Evelyn Unes-Hansen for contributing her expertise to this book. Thanks to Dr. William Timmons for his dedication to this field and for sharing his knowledge with me. Thanks to my sister Anjie, whom I love dearly. Very special thanks to Jim Sarno, Jess Altimarano, and Sue and Diamond Sloan—these people have all been a part of my becoming what I am today. Their contributions to the fabric that makes my persona were significant and worthwhile.

And thanks to Andrew Steinberg, Mel Berger, Arnold Rifkin, Dana Isaacson, and Judith Regan for making the dream a reality.

INTRODUCTION

"*P*roper diet" continues to elude us. As a nation, we are fatter and more unhealthy than ever before, even though we have more people dieting and exercising here than anywhere else in the world and more than anytime in our history. We cannot get it right. Is the proper diet high in carbohydrates? Low in fat? High, or low in protein? What is it? Help!

The reason that proper diet is so elusive is quite simple:

There is no proper diet!

Each individual has a unique metabolism. The inner workings of each and every person's metabolism are vastly different. It is because of these differences that it is impossible for one way of eating to work for everyone.

There have been many great diet books written by many great authors, and all of these books all have valuable information that may work for many people. But these diet books are facing an impossible task: To address the needs of different types of metabolisms with only one approach—it doesn't work that way.

Even in medical school, our very best doctors are taught that we are all basically the same. They are taught that with minor exceptions, we all share the same physiology and chemistry and homeostatic internal environment. I am here to tell you that that is far from the truth. We are all different. We all have unique and ever-changing internal environments—we are homeodynamic.

I have written this book to put an end to the confusion.

This book was written not for the scientist, but for the layman, and for this reason, I have kept it as simple as possible. This book was written to empower the individual who is faced with so many choices, and so many conflicting opinions. Finally, that individual will be able to cut through all the misinformation and clutter that has become the diet industry, and arrive at a profound perspective and solutions to their personal dilemma. This book will direct the individual to a nutritional program designed specifically for his or her unique needs. Fulfilling those unique needs will facilitate tremendous changes to the individual's appearance, vitality, stamina, and overall health and wellness.

HOLLYWOOD'S
healthiest
diets

IT'S ALL ABOUT FAT

Counting calories and fat grams, and weighing ourselves, has made us the fattest nation on the planet

WITHIN A MONTH, YOU WILL BE SHOCKED WHEN YOU LOOK IN THE MIRROR

*T*hese first four chapters will enable you to understand the physical transformation you will be experiencing. These chapters provide a detailed explanation of how to make it possible for your body to burn the fat off, *and you will learn to keep it off.* This book is a state-of-the-art roadmap to losing fat, weight, and inches. When you are on this path, you will definitely lose unwanted body-fat. You will not experience parts of the day when your energy crashes. Your health, especially your immune system, will be working at its fullest capacity, and you will feel better than you've ever felt. Within these pages you will *finally* discover how to train your metabolism to work at its fullest possible capacity, and *you will teach your metabolism to work at this optimal level forever.*

I will give you the exact same information that I gave to Demi Moore, to transform her body for *Striptease* and *G.I. Jane.* You will discover how Paula Abdul attained the beautiful physique she has today. You will learn how Angela Bassett and Vincent Spano look and feel their best, how Robin Williams was able to shed inches from his waistline, and how Bruce Willis and Denzel Washington maintain their athletic appearance. Because you will find the program that is perfect for your unique metabolism, you will get the results you desire. You will train your metabolism to work like it's on fire. You will be energized from the moment you wake up until bedtime. You will be more capable of handling stress. You will not get sick as often. You will think more clearly. You will find these nutritional programs to work better than liposuction, reducing your body-fat in a dramatic and *lasting* fashion.

WEIGHT LOSS VS. BODY-FAT REDUCTION

When people come to my clinic to see me, they have many of the same thoughts you had when you bought this book. They come in saying, "I want to lose weight." Weight is not the issue. Your weight on the scale has nothing—*absolutely nothing*—to do with the problem.

"O.K., I'm too fat and I want to lose weight." This is an oxymoron. Is it *weight* you want to lose or is it *fat* you want to lose? Do you want to lose muscle that burns calories making the metabolism work more efficiently, powering the immune system, preventing osteoporosis? Is it water weight that you want to lose? (Water that will return as soon as you eat normally again.) Is it much needed bone tissue that should be wasted away? The answer is a resounding *no*. The issue is not weight. The issue is *body-fat*.

The simple truth is that you are too fat. It took me a long time to say this to my patients. I would try to pad or sweeten the way I said it, but after some time, I found that my clients actually appreciated me saying it. More often than not, my clients say, "That makes so much sense. Why hasn't anyone ever said that to me before?"

We are too fat, and as a result, some of us are also too heavy.

You wake up. Within thirty minutes you are on the scale weighing yourself. It is the same routine for many millions of Americans. People are weighing themselves because of a misconception that weight indicates *fatness*. Anyone who is dieting in an effort to lose "weight" is actually interested in the reduction of body-fat. It is the fat that makes us too large. It is the fat that makes us too heavy.

> ### *Weighing ourselves is the misleading manner by which we gauge* how fat we are.

Americans have been "watching their weight" for many years. In fact, many millions have watched it go down and back up many times. We have grown to view the scale as the barometer of our appearance. In reality, the scale has nothing to do with the way we look. The only reason we use the scale is that it is the only way that we have been able to check our progress in the "war on weight."

Last year Americans spent more than $9 billion on *weight loss*. This is more than the gross national product of over 50% of the countries in the world. This staggering figure *does not* include apparel, all the gym memberships, and the array of products attached to the **fitness industry**. We are talking about money that was paid to somebody or some place or for special foods to lose "weight," for nutritional supplements, diet drugs, special gadgets, etc. This year there are more people on diets than ever before. This year there are more people *gaining weight* than at any other time in history. In this country there are more people paying attention to fat grams, and partaking in fat-free diets than anywhere else in the world, and at the same time we have more fat people per capita than any other country. We have more fat people this year than last year, which was more than the year before that. Clearly the issue isn't weight loss. If it were, everyone would be skinny.

I urge you to go to your local diet outlet, stand outside like a researcher, and simply ask the people coming in if they have been on that diet system in the past. Then ask them how many times. The fact is that all these diet franchises share one business trait:

> ### *All are sustained in large part on repeat business, and have few new customers.*

It isn't the person returning for the umpteenth time to lose weight who is at fault. It is the manner in which they lost the weight. The majority of the weight they lost was bone, muscle and organ weight, water, and *very little body-fat. The human body, which has been designed to survive, will replace those important tissues as soon as possible with some additional fat.* Statistics show that persons who go on typical low calorie diets will regain 107% of the weight. This is what is commonly referred to as a syndrome called yo-yo-dieting. Don't you agree that it is time to stop this ridiculous cycle?

When I look at myself in the morning for my daily assessment, I do not guess at how much I weigh; I simply say, "Am I too fat or not?" To varying degrees, it's the same thing we all do, but somewhere along the way, it got translated into pounds. When you weigh yourself on the scale, you weigh your whole body, *not how much fat you have.* You weigh your hair, your bones, your teeth, your muscles, your organs, and so on. **In no way does your body-weight reflect how fat you are.** A loss of a pound may indicate less food in your stomach, less water retention than yesterday. It may be the loss of a pound of muscle because you starved yourself. It certainly does not mean you are any less fat.

You picked up this book because you do not want to be fat. So get rid of the entire notion of "watching your weight." At no time, from this moment forward, will your weight on the scale give any indication of your progress or be a method to gauge your results. What you have to focus on is this: **"How much of my body is fat?"** and **"How do I reduce that amount of fat?"**

That is exactly what we will discuss in this book—It is exactly the information you are craving—*The process of fat reduction, not* **weight reduction.** Keep in mind that you will actually lose pounds, but the number of pounds you lose will not necessarily correlate with the changes you see in the mirror. At no time will your weight on the scale reflect what is really happening to your body. There will be times when you are certain that you are leaner or smaller, and yet the scale may say that you did not lose an ounce. You will have many ways to gauge your progress, but your weight on the scale is not one of them. You will continually be seeing improvements in your appearance. You will see changes in the way your clothes fit, you will be in a smaller size, feel much lighter, harder, and look much healthier.

Muscle and bone density increases will affect your weight.

There are many reasons not to trust your scale. When on any of the ten nutritional programs contained within these covers, you will be achieving results that your scale cannot decipher. The increase in muscle and bone density you will experience will affect your weight on the scale. Muscle and bone density *decrease* over time for many reasons. These reasons include dieting, lack of activity, age, hormonal imbalances, and usage of certain drugs. For example, as one follows a typical low calorie "diet," the body will use the protein in its muscles to survive. Because muscle is very heavy, this reduction of muscle tissue causes a big drop in weight.

Keep in mind that the muscles in our bodies burn calories all day—even while we are at rest. In fact, 75% of all the energy burned in a day is burned while we are at rest. So, as unknowing dieters lose "weight," they are often losing muscle, decreasing the body's ability to burn off calories and insuring that they will always be "battling the bulge."

Muscle creates a firmer, tighter appearance; it fuels the metabolism, and it makes us strong and energetic. Lack of muscle leaves a person soft and "squishy," weak, lethargic, prone to osteoporosis, and guarantees *a sluggish metabolism*. By following the appropriate plan within this book, you will be able to *restore* muscle that you have lost on other "diets." By rebuilding this lost tissue, you will be able to burn many more calories each day—which translates into faster, easier fat loss. By adding this muscle, you will gain a firmer, harder appearance. You will also have much more energy. Keep in mind that we are talking about increasing the *density* of your muscles. The size of your muscles will not increase. This increase in muscle density may adversely affect your weight. As you lose the fat, you will be replacing it with muscle and bone.

Another negative aspect of typical low calorie diets is that they are almost always *low nutrient* diets. Because the bones in your body require nutrients, they will often lose density when on reduced calorie and nutrient intake. While following any nutritional program in this book, you will have adequate levels of nutrient intake, which will allow your bones to regain lost density. Again, this increase in bone density will not make your body any larger, but will offset some of your weight loss, because some of the fat-weight will be replaced by bone-weight.

If I can't weigh myself, how will I know if it's working?

The most accurate way to chart your progress while on any diet is to measure the amount of fat in your body. This is *to figure out how many pounds of fat you have.* This is called determining your body-fat percentage.

Here's an example: Lisa wants to find a more accurate way to check her progress while on a new nutritional program. Basically what she wants is a "before and after" picture that is much more accurate and representative of her achievements than the scale would be. She wants to learn two things: how much of her weight on the scale is fat (the bad stuff), and how much of her weight is muscle, bone, organs, etc. (the good stuff).

Lisa gets on the scale and finds that she weighs 168 pounds. **Because she has had her body-fat measured,** Lisa knows that she has 34% body-fat. This means that 34% of her weight on the scale is fat. She uses a simple calculation to determine how many pounds of fat she is carrying around.

168 lbs. × 34% body-fat = 57.1 lbs. of fat

She uses a similar calculation to determine how much lean body mass (the good stuff) she has working for her.

168 lbs. − 57.1 lbs. of fat = 110.9 lbs. of lean body mass (muscle, bones, organs, etc.)

Lisa then follows the nutritional program that is most appropriate for her. She follows the program for 30 days. She feels leaner, her energy is high, and she is feeling healthier than when she started. She steps on the scale, and to her surprise, she has lost very little weight (only three pounds). Thankfully, she has read this chapter of the book and will not be discouraged by what she is seeing on the scale, because she knows there is much more to the story. Instead of becoming discouraged, she gets a more accurate picture of what is happening. **She has her body-fat measured again,** and to her delight, she is now at 31% body-fat.

165 lbs. × 31% body-fat = 51.1 lbs. of fat.

This means she has lost 6 pounds of fat, even though she still weighs 165 pounds. This was due to an increase of the density of her muscles and bones of 3 pounds. Her body is smaller, leaner, and better looking, but weighs nearly the same.

On the other hand, she could have gone to the corner diet center and followed the wrong kind of diet and had the following (and very typical) results: She starts at the same point (168 pounds with 34% body-fat = 57.1 pounds of fat) and she has working in her favor 110.9 pounds of muscles, bones, organs, etc. She stays on the program, she fights her food cravings, and she is determined to really lose some weight. When she returns to the diet center she is weighed, and she is ecstatic with her achievement. She now weighs 158 pounds on the scale! Wow, she lost 10 pounds!

But if she was determined to lose body-fat, and had that body-fat measured, she would have discovered that her loss was more of a defeat than it was a victory. She would have found that her body-fat was close to 34%. That means that she still had 53.7 pounds of fat—a loss of only 3.4 pounds of fat. More importantly she would realize that she now had only 104.3 lbs. of muscles, bones, organs, etc. (the good stuff)—**a loss of *6.6 lbs. of the wrong stuff!***

WHAT IS FAT, AND WHAT DOES FAT DO?

Insulation

Fat is absolutely essential to our health and wellness, and performs many vital functions in the body. One of the many functions body-fat serves in our bodies is as insulation. *You do require* a small amount of body-fat, called subcutaneous fat, which is located directly under the skin, to maintain a normal body temperature. Without a small amount of body-fat, one could not maintain normal body temperatures, and if it were 70 degrees outside we would, in time, freeze to death. So yes, a small amount of subcutaneous (under the skin) body-fat is required to maintain your survival. When I say small amount, I mean that if you pinch the skin on the inside of your forearm, you will see approximately the amount of this type of fat that is essential.

Hormonal Balance

Another function that fat serves in the body is to maintain a normal hormonal balance. This is especially true in women. Certain hormones are carried and stored within fat cells to be brought back into the bloodstream and called back into service. It is not uncommon that, when large amounts of fat reduction occur, blood levels of many hormones can be well above, and below "normal."

ORGAN SUPPORT

Fat serves to maintain precise organ positioning within the body, and especially, in the abdominal and chest cavity. This is called visceral fat. There is also fat in and around the brain.

Fat helps to stabilize muscles and joints to keep them in their proper positions. Fat also facilitates normal nervous system function. Nerves can sometimes travel through a very thin layer of fat tissue to protect themselves. Fat also provides a way that the body can detoxify itself. Excessive amounts of chemicals, pesticides, and hormones from exterior sources will be removed from the bloodstream and stored in fat cells, to be passed through the system when it is not overburdened.

The number of fat cells that a person has will have been determined by the end of puberty, and that is the number of fat cells that you will have for the rest of you life—that is all you will ever have. So there are a finite number of fat cells in your body; however, the ability of each fat cell to shrink or grow is nearly infinite. Each fat cell can be reduced to about $\frac{1}{1000}$ the diameter of a human hair. Conversely, a fat cell can expand to about the size of a baseball.

FAT AND STARVATION

The most important knowledge for our purpose is that fat serves as a storage place for energy or calories. This storage system is key to our survival; if we were truly starving, the body would call on this calorie storage reserve to feed itself. One pound of body-fat contains about 3,500 calories, and most persons can survive at a basal rate (that is to say, remaining relatively still—without exercising, expending large amounts of energy, or enduring extremely cold temperatures) on as little as 400 calories a day. Meaning that one pound of fat can sustain us without food for many days. Unfortunately, we can't just starve ourselves to reduce the level of body-fat. In such extreme survival conditions, the body will burn other tissues in addition to burning fat. First, the body will deplete its stored sugar. This stored sugar is called glycogen. When glycogen is gone, the body will begin consuming its own muscle and organs. Fat stores are called on last, as the body realizes that when the fat is totally gone, so are you. Whereas the body will only call upon its fat reserve when faced with imminent death, eliminating muscle and organ tissue does not mean imminent death to the body.

METHODS OF BODY-FAT MEASUREMENT

There are quite a few ways to have your body-fat measured. These methods range from inexpensive to prohibitively costly and from fairly accurate to scientifically exact. Some methods require assistance of a trained professional, while others can be done at home alone.

The most convenient method is called bio-impedance. For this procedure, one would either hold onto metal bars or electrodes attached by adhesive to the hand and foot, and a weak, undetectable current of electricity is passed through your body. The resistance that the electricity is met by can be measured and scientific calculations can be applied to determine how much of your total weight is comprised of fat. Body-fat provides a different resistance to electricity than muscle, water or bone. When you do choose this method, you must maintain *exactly* the same level of physical activity, and dietary intake for each 24-hour period directly preceding the test. When you are able to accomplish this, the accuracy of this test can be as close as plus or minus 1%.

There are home machines on the market that can be purchased at a fairly reasonable price. The Tanita Corporation (1–800–9–TANITA) has made great strides in developing affordable and accurate instruments that are definitely the finest products available. The product is built into a precision scale, as bodyweight is a necessary factor in determining your body-fat percentage. Because the Tanita scale represents the most convenient method to track and monitor your progress over time, it is definitely recommended *in this class*.

Another method to measure body-fat percentage is the skin-fold caliper technique. The skin-fold caliper is a device that measures the thickness of the layer of fat, by pinching a fold of skin and fat between the index finger and thumb, and then measuring the thickness of this fold with the device. These measurements are taken in different places on the body.

The most accurate formula when using the skin-fold caliper is a four-site measurement. The measurements are taken at the back of the triceps, two inches to the left of the belly button, on your waistline just above the crest of your pelvic bone (called the superiliac crest), and the front of your thigh. All of these measurements are taken on the left side. When skin-fold calipers are used appropriately by a trained clinician, the accuracy factor is about plus or minus 2%, which is a fairly accurate measurement. Because the measurements are taken in various locations on the body, you will be able to get a much better idea of where you are or where you are *not* losing body fat. As you identify problem areas, changes and/or additional supplementation may be implemented to more effectively treat and produce a positive response in these areas of the body. (See Yohimbe, Chapter 5).

There are several other methods that are too expensive, too inaccurate, or too obscure to make them worth your time and energy. I will list a few so that you can save yourself the aggrava-tion. One of these methods of body-fat measurement is called the BodPod. This egg-shaped apparatus costs close to $30,000 and one should expect this measurement to cost roughly $50 per session. Another method of measurement is called hydrostatic weighing. Performed by an experienced team of professionals, the cost of this test is usually over $200 per session. Dual X-ray absorptiometry is a very specialized procedure performed in only a handful of loca-tions around the world like NASA, and will cost about $500 per visit. So this is probably not an option for you. Another expensive and hard-to-find option is called spectroscopy. This method is extremely accurate and very expensive, costing up to $2500 per ses-sion. The least accurate way to measure body-fat is called Body Mass Index, where certain measurements are taken, such as the cir-cumference of your waist, arm, etc., and from those measurements a formula to determine your body-fat percentage is calculated. I would not recommend this, and have found it to be extremely unreliable.

Again, you don't need to shell out thousands of dollars. Look in the mirror. Feel how your slacks fit. Pinch your love handles. You will be absolutely certain when you are achieving results.

If you want to have a tangible and clear picture of those results, **I recommend that you measure your body-fat percentage at least once per month**. When using a home bio-impedance machine, you may choose to measure more frequently based upon your needs. If you choose to have a clinician take this measurement, you should have the same person take the measurement, using the same instruments, at the same location, and when possible it should be at the same time of the day. You want to make the conditions as favorable as possible to have the measurement be as accurate as it can be.

Chart 01.01

Body-fat Chart for Females

Obese	=	Above 28%
Acceptable	=	Below 28%
Fit	=	Below 20%
Lean	=	Below 18%
Very lean	=	Below 14%
Unsafe	=	Below 10%

Body-fat Chart for Males

Obese	=	Above 26%
Acceptable	=	Below 23%
Fit	=	Below 18%
Lean	=	Below 14%
Very lean	=	Below 10%
Unsafe	=	Below 4%

THE RIGHT FOOD AT THE RIGHT TIME

*The building-blocks to your
physical transformation*

YOU ARE NOT ALONE

*I*f you are like most people, you have tried dieting before. Dieting has become an obsession. You cannot turn on the television, open a newspaper, or walk through the checkout line at the grocery store without being bombarded by the latest dieting craze. Dieting is now a multi-billion dollar industry, and more often than not, that multi-billion dollar industry perpetuates myths that make you fatter than you were before you began your diet.

Have you ever wondered why even though you do not overeat, you continue to gain weight? Have you been frustrated by the perpetual diet cycle? Are you always watching what you eat, but never seeing any results? Do you wonder why you get severe food cravings and crippling hunger when you try to follow any kind of strict dietary regimen? Why is it that you exercise like crazy, but do not see any significant change in your appearance? Have you noticed that eating the same old way is now making you fatter? Do you have severe drops in your energy levels at certain times during the day? *All of these scenarios are the results of the exact same problem.* The information in this chapter will get a bit technical, but I will make it easy enough for you to understand. It is important—no, it is absolutely essential for you to have this knowledge, so take a few minutes to read through this chapter. I promise it will be worth your time.

In this chapter, you will be given the scientific basis and philosophy for the nutritional programs contained in this book. In the first chapter, we discussed the difference between weight loss and fat reduction. In this chapter, you will learn what is actually happening when you reduce the amount of fat in your body, and more importantly how to reduce your percentage of body-fat.

There is only one way to reduce your percentage of fat: *eat the right foods at the right times.* Easy to say, but what the right foods are, and what the right time is, will be vastly different for each individual. The question is: "What are the right foods, and the right times for you?" That is the big question. To answer this question for yourself, there are some key factors to consider. In this chapter, I will discuss some primary considerations of fat loss. Specifically, calories, metabolism, food choices, and how to combine foods in the proper way to get the results you want. To understand what the right food and what the right time is for you, each of these key issues will be discussed separately. Understanding these issues will be the basis of your physical transformation. In the process, I hope that we can dispel some myths that the diet industry has led you to believe, and give you a comprehensive understanding of the changes you will be seeing in your mirror.

CALORIE COUNTING IS NOT THE ANSWER

One of the first pieces of misinformation that was perpetrated on the public by the diet industry was that you only had to watch your calories. The supposition was that if you burned more calories than you consumed, then weight loss would occur. While that might be true, it does not mean that the weight that would be lost would be fat. Until recently, scientists were convinced that all calories were created equal. It has always been said that "a calorie is a calorie." Nothing could be further from the truth. Calories are definitely not the most important issue in any fat reduction plan. They are only one important part of the puzzle.

A calorie is simply a measurement of the amount of literal energy contained in a portion of food. One calorie is the amount of energy required to raise the temperature of one cubic centimeter of water by one degree. All foods have calories. Proteins have 4.2 calories per gram by weight. Carbohydrates also have 4.2 calories per gram. Fat has 9.4 calories per gram. Everyone's body has a need for calories on an ongoing basis. Every activity a person engages in, even watching television, burns calories. Just sitting still burns calories. In fact, on average, 75% of all the calories burned by the average person in a day are burned while at rest. Certain activities cause an increased rate of calorie burning, hence the idea that repetitive exercise is essential to body-fat loss. This however, is also a myth. For example, jogging for an hour will burn several hundred calories, but just sitting still in water that is below 60 degrees Fahrenheit will burn many more.

Unfortunately, it is nearly impossible for you to determine an exact caloric value of food. By placing a food in a special machine called a calorimeter, the actual amount of caloric energy within that food can be measured. The machine works by burning the food and measuring the amount of heat produced. Unfortunately, the human body is not a furnace and does not burn food. It must slowly digest and process and assimilate food. In addition to variations in the ways each individual processes and assimilates those foods, there are numerous other factors that make it very difficult to determine the actual caloric value of a food. These variables include the following:

1. *The thermic effect of food.* This is the amount of calories that the body will burn while digesting and processing this food.

2. *The amount of fiber.* How many of the calories contained in this food are coming from fiber? Fiber is nondigestible, so, even though it may contain energy, your body cannot use it.

3. *The digestibility of the food.* Certain foods are not well digested, especially in persons who have digestive dysfunction. Even though the foods have calories, some will pass through the body undigested.

What you really want to do is to reduce the amount of fat on your body, right? *Calorie counting is not the **key** to that fat reduction,* **it is only a part of the total equation**. Many different companies within the diet industry suggest that you should only have so many calories in any given day. The truth is, that number is different for everyone. The number of calories consumed on any one of the ten food plans in this book can vary by several hundred per day. As you will learn in this chapter, it is not the total number of calories, but the ratio of protein, carbohydrates and fats, that paves your road to leanness.

PROTEINS, FATS, AND CARBOHYDRATES

What They Are and How They Work

Now that you have a basic understanding of calories and their relative unimportance with regard to fat loss, let's look at where these calories come from—food. What you are trying to determine is: "What is the right food, and what is the right time for me?" To answer that question will require that we have some information about the foods that you will be eating. Any food will fall into one of three categories: **proteins, carbohydrates, and fats**.

PROTEIN

The Building Blocks of the Human Body

For those of you who have lost several pounds, only to find that it is impossible to keep them off for a long period, this information will be a revelation. The cause of this phenomenon is simple.

When you lost the weight, you were not losing just fat. Because the diet you were following was deficient in protein, relative to your individual needs for protein, some or much of the weight you were losing was from muscle and the other protein-based tissues in your body. This loss of protein-based tissue causes a "slowing" of the metabolism, by creating imbalances in certain hormones. Over time you would have to eat smaller and smaller portions of food because your body is unable to burn off the normal amount of calories. Over time, you will have a higher and higher percentage of body-fat, even though your total bodyweight is lower.

You *must* derive the adequate amount of protein from your diet or suffer. Suffer what? Lowered energy, weakened immune response, weaker bones, skin problems, hair loss at an early age, hormonal imbalances, high cholesterol, liver toxicity, premature aging. . . . The list goes on and on.

Protein is essential and you must have it with every meal—every day.

The large majority of your entire body is protein. If all of the water were removed from your body, 80% of what remained would be comprised of protein. Your hair is protein; your nails have protein in them; skin, heart, liver, kidneys, bones, brain, and all other parts of your body contain protein. These tissues must be maintained properly in order to remain in optimal wellness. Their maintenance requires an adequate intake of protein from the diet. Failure to consume adequate dietary protein guarantees that you will never enjoy optimal wellness or appearance.

Protein has 4.2 calories per gram, by weight. Scientifically speaking, proteins are amino acids that are linked together by peptide bonds in a chain that is referred to as a protein chain, or, a protein. Think of amino acids as the beads in a necklace. When the beads are sitting on a surface, they are just beads. When the beads are linked together by a strand, they become jewelry. When individual amino acids link together, they become proteins. Amino acids exist in nature in every form of life. There are hundreds of different amino acids. The human body needs 22 specific amino acids to survive. Of those 22 amino acids, the body can only produce 11. The other 11 are what are called "essential amino acids." The term "essential" means that they must be supplied in adequate amounts by the diet, or a deficiency disease will result.

When there is an insufficient amount of protein in your diet, your body will use the protein from its own tissues to satisfy its physiological needs. In other words, your body will cannibalize its own tissues—muscle, organs, tendons, ligaments, etc.—in order to get the protein it needs. When there is a protein deficiency, the first tissue to be sacrificed is muscle. Muscle is needed to burn calories, make us strong, shapely, and energetic. When you lose muscle, you lose the ability to burn calories. In other words, when you don't eat enough protein, you slow down the metabolism, weaken the body, and lower your energy levels.

The quality of the protein is an important factor.

When you follow any of the nutritional programs in this book, your protein will come from foods such as chicken, turkey, fish, egg whites, beef, veal, lamb, venison, soy products, low-fat or non-fat cheese and cottage cheese, protein powders, etc. Although foods such as beans, legumes, nuts, grains, and yogurt have some proteins, they also contain many carbohydrates and fats, and the protein quality of these foods is very low. The quality of protein is really a measurement of how efficiently the body is able to assimilate and use the protein. There are two major methods for determining the quality of a protein.

The most reliable measurement of protein quality for our purposes is what is known as the biological value. The biological value, known as the BV, is a number assigned to a protein food to indicate three major factors about the protein:

1. How easy the protein is for the body to digest.
2. How well the protein matches the types of proteins found in the body.
3. How fast protein is absorbed into the cells of the body.

Table 02.01

The following is a list of the biological value (BV) of a few selected proteins:

- Whey protein (partially predigested, ion exchanged, microfiltered)   130+
- Egg white   104
- Chicken breast   84
- Beef   78
- Soy protein   74
- Milk protein   72
- Fish (average)   75
- Beans   45
- Nuts   40

While trying to reduce the amount of fat in your body, it will be of significant benefit to you to consume proteins with the highest BV, as these proteins will have the most benefit to your body.

Each individual has a unique requirement for protein. How much is enough? After answering the questions contained in Chapter 6, "Is This You?" of this book, you will discover that one or more nutritional programs are appropriate for you. When you choose the diet that is the best fit, you will be led though a process to determine your exact needs. There will be your answer.

FAT

Everyone knows what fat is:

- Fat is butter.
- Fat is oil.
- Fat is lard. Fat is what hangs around your middle.
- Fat is why you bought this book.

Scientifically, fat is composed of three fatty acids bonded to a glycerol molecule. Fat is not a substance to be feared or hated. Fat is absolutely essential for human survival, and your failure to consume enough of it guarantees your failure as a dieter. Fat is something the body stores for energy on reserve. Fat gives women a different appearance than it gives men. Fat helps the nervous system function. Fat holds the organs of the body in their correct places. Fat insulates the body. Fat is in just about every cell in the body, and it performs a wide array of functions. Fat is essential to your health and critical to your success as a dieter.

There are many different sources of fat in the diet. It is nearly impossible to avoid fat, as it is in almost every food. Foods such as oils, butter, nuts, full fat cheeses, avocados, olives, certain cuts of meats, are very high in fat. Foods such as fruit, vegetables, most grains, potatoes, and others are very low in fat. Very few foods have no fat at all. The exceptions to this are man-made foods that have been manipulated so as not to contain fat.

There are different types of fats, too. There are good fats and bad fats. Good fats, or unsaturated fats, are beneficial to the body in a number of ways, and should be sought after. These good fats are found in such foods as olives, avocados, olive oil, safflower oil, flax oil, nuts, etc. Bad fats, or saturated fats, are the kinds of fats that clog the arteries, make cholesterol levels rise, and may raise blood pressure. Bad fats are found in such foods as meats, cheeses, butter, lard, and cream. Although you will be allowed to consume some of the bad fats, you should always try to keep the majority of your fat intake coming from the good fats.

Fat Is Not the Enemy

Contrary to very popular belief, fat is not the enemy of dieters. In fact, fat is actually the least fattening of all the food types. Although fat has twice as many calories as the other food types, fat does not stimulate significant production of insulin, which is the body's fat-making hormone. (Insulin will be discussed later in this chapter.) Fat can actually stop other foods from making you fat by inhibiting the digestion of these foods and the subsequent release of the digested foods into the bloodstream. The more slowly food that you have eaten is absorbed into the bloodstream, the less likely it is to be turned to fat. Fat can also help you lose fat because it is very satiating. Fat makes you feel full and satisfied, making it less likely that you will overeat. *The trick with fat, as with all the food types, is to determine how much, and when, you need it.*

One thing is for certain. You definitely need at least some fat. You must never try to be on a fat-free diet. Eating fat-free foods is not the answer. In fact, eating fat-free guarantees that you will always have too much of it under your skin. Once you have located the correct diet in this book, you will learn what the right amount of fat is for you.

CARBOHYDRATES

Carbohydrate balance is critical to achieving lasting fat loss. Carbohydrates should never have been called carbohydrates. They are sugar. No matter how complex, carbohydrates are broken down to their lowest common denominator, which is glucose. Glucose is sugar. Carbohydrates are your body's primary fuel source. Your brain requires carbohydrates every second of its life. Carbohydrates, in the form of blood sugar, are pumping through your veins every minute of the day. And while they are essential to your survival, they can also be your worst enemy. The most difficult part of finding the right diet will be in determining the correct amount of carbohydrates.

Carbohydrates are found in the diet in many places. Sources of carbohydrates include fruit, flour, breads, yams, potatoes, rice, oatmeal, beans, and so on. Scientifically, a carbohydrate is a molecule made of two or more carbon atoms bonded with hydrogen and oxygen. There are different types of carbohydrates as well. There are simple-, medium-, and long-chain (complex) carbohydrates. Simple carbohydrates are very easy for the body to break down and absorb, because their chemical structure is very simple. Medium-chain carbohydrates are slightly more detailed in their structure and will take longer for the body to digest and absorb, leading to a longer-lasting release of energy. Complex carbohydrates are very intricately-assembled molecules and are the most difficult to be broken down and utilized by the body, resulting in a long-lasting release of energy.

The body's primary fuel is glucose. Glucose is a simple carbohydrate, also known as a sugar. This sugar controls many functions in the body and must be carefully balanced to achieve wellness and lasting fat loss. One common goal of all ten diets in this book is to control the level of glucose in the bloodstream. The stabilization of glucose is essential. Glucose levels will be the final determinant in the war on fat. When glucose levels are too high, all of the body's functions will suffer, just as they will when glucose levels are too low. The amount and type of carbohydrates being ingested will have significant impact on the levels of glucose within the blood. Correctly balancing the amount and types of carbohydrates you are consuming will have enormous impact on the level of fat in your body.

Carbohydrates are actually the most fattening of all the food types, because they have the highest potential to cause imbalances in the body's sugar levels and the body's hormones, especially insulin. (Hormones are discussed later in this chapter.) The imbalances in hormones that result from the improper types and amounts of carbohydrates can stop fat loss cold and create a favorable environment for diseases of various types.

All ten diets within this book share one common goal—to carefully regulate the amount of glucose in the bloodstream of the person who is following the plan. Some people need a lot of carbohydrates to regulate glucose, while other people must eliminate nearly all carbohydrates from their diets, because their bodies have learned how to make all the sugar they need from other foods.

YOUR METABOLISM

When people hear the word "metabolism," they think of some system in the body that burns the calories they eat. You may have heard people say that they have a "slow" or a "fast" metabolism.

The notion that you can have a fast or slow metabolism is actually another myth. Metabolism refers to the *way*, not the speed at which your body processes and utilizes the food and nutrients you eat each day. This process does not happen faster or slower, just differently, for each individual. The metabolism is really the cumulative effect of certain hormones in your body. It is the goal of this book to teach you to eat in such a way as to bring balance back to your hormones. In doing so, you will achieve an optimal appearance and top physical health. Correct combinations of food are the only way to achieve this balance.

When there is an *imbalance* in the hormones that make up your metabolism, your personal health problems lurk right around the corner. Hormonal imbalances will not only prevent the reduction of body-fat, but will also stimulate the *accumulation* of body-fat, and all too often, these hormonal imbalances are also the root of many disease states. Diseases such as diabetes, high blood pressure, the various forms of cardiovascular disease, stroke, aneurysm, cancer of various kinds, dementia, osteoporosis, certain forms of arthritis, chronic depression, anxiety, insomnia, and many others are caused, at least in part, by hormonal imbalances. Many medical reports in the recent past have even attributed schizophrenia to dietary-related hormonal imbalance.

THE BIG FOUR

The hormones that are doing most of the work in your metabolism are insulin, cortisol, glucagon, and human growth hormone (HGH). There are literally a hundred others at work, but as far as metabolism goes, they all play roles of lesser importance. Let's take a brief look at the "big four" and what they do for your body.

INSULIN

Your Best Friend and Worst Enemy

Insulin has two absolutely critical roles in the body, two functions that we cannot live without, and yet insulin can also be the root of your demise. Insulin's first function in the body is to carry sugar (glucose), fat, and protein into your cells where they can be used for energy and repair. Most of all, all of the trillions of cells in your body need glucose and/or protein to survive, and insulin is how they get it. Insulin, secreted by the pancreas, attaches itself to these molecules and transports them out of the blood and into the various cells of the body.

When you eat, a certain amount of the food will be converted into glucose and enter the bloodstream. As the sugar level rises, the body senses it and secretes insulin to lower the sugar. This is insulin's second main function in the body—to lower glucose levels. If you eat too much of any food, especially carbohydrates, the levels of glucose in the blood rise to very high levels. In turn, this triggers a large release of insulin from the pancreas. Insulin will proceed to put the available glucose, fat, and protein away into your body's muscle, organ and brain cells, where it can be used for the production of energy and for the repair of the cells.

If your cells do not need *all* of the glucose, fat, and protein *right at that moment*, insulin will begin the process of converting the extra food into fat and then put it all away into your *fat cells*. Because insulin can so quickly turn and become the arch-enemy of fat reduction, you must gain an understanding of this hormone and do all in your power to keep it under control. By combining foods appropriately for your body, you will maintain optimum levels of insulin throughout the day.

GLUCAGON

Insulin's Counterpart

Glucagon is the antithesis of insulin. Its main job in the body is to raise the blood glucose level when it is too low. Insulin and glucagon must be in equilibrium for you to enjoy wellness and fat reduction. When glucagon levels are normal, the body will use the sugar from the blood to fuel itself. When glucagon levels rise too high, usually because of undereating, the brain can initiate a process called gluconeogenesis—the creation of sugar from protein.

This is what often happens to people when they go on "diets" that are very low in calories. The low sugar levels in the blood force the levels of glucagon to skyrocket, and this leads to the loss of muscle and other protein tissues, because the body is trying to make sugar from them.

When glucagon is too low, it cannot oppose the functions of insulin, and the level of glucose can fall sharply. This condition is called hypoglycemia. When sugar levels are too low, your energy will also be low. When sugar levels are too low, the body will sense it as starvation and shut down fat burning. The body will hold onto its fat reserve until the very last moment—after all the muscles and other protein tissues have wasted away. Glucagon management is accomplished by maintaining normal glucose levels in the blood. This is achieved by eating the right food at the right time.

CORTISOL

The Potentially Evil Stress Hormone

Cortisol is produced by the adrenal glands, two peanut-shaped glands that sit just above the kidneys, deep in the abdominal cavity. Cortisol is a hormone that is needed by the body for normal immune system function, regulation of blood pressure, regulation of inflammation, and many other things. Cortisol can also be extremely deadly. Have you ever heard the saying "stress kills"? Well, the saying should really be that cortisol kills. During times of stress, cortisol is elevated. High levels of cortisol are known to be a cause of decreased bone density, increased blood pressure, inhibition of the immune system, muscle wasting, insulin resistance, and certainly a main cause of increased body-fat levels. In addition to stress, there are other factors that can elevate cortisol. Significant fluctuations in blood sugar can elevate cortisol. Excessive carbohydrates relative to your needs will elevate cortisol. Protein deficiency can elevate it. Even eating too little can cause cortisol to rise.

Cortisol is able to overpower just about all other hormones in the body. It will raise glucose even when insulin is trying to lower it. Cortisol can lower glucose in the presence of glucagon. It can cause accumulation of body-fat even if you are doing just about everything correctly. Cortisol will block HGH from doing its job. (See HGH discussed below.)

The proper level of cortisol is achieved through proper combinations of food, relative to your needs. By mixing the right amounts of the right foods at the right times, you can bring about an optimal level of cortisol.

HUMAN GROWTH HORMONE

The Hormone That Does It All

Human growth hormone, known as HGH, is secreted by the pituitary gland, a small gland that sits directly behind the eyes at the front of the brain. HGH has many benefits to the body and virtually no negative effects. It is one of the goals of this book to teach you to eat and behave in such a way that would maximize the amount of HGH in your bloodstream at all times.

HGH increases lean body mass. In other words, it increases the amount of protein tissues in the body—muscle. HGH decreases body-fat. HGH increases memory, stamina, libido and normalizes blood pressure. HGH increases the effectiveness of the immune system. Low levels of HGH can cause anxiety, depression, aggressive aging, low energy levels and increased body-fat. Low levels of HGH can cause a weakening of the immune system, which can lead to all sorts of diseases ranging from cancer to diabetes.

HGH is produced in large amounts when we are young and begins to decline as we age. By the time an adult has reached fifty years of age, the level of HGH in their blood has fallen by at least 40%. The decline in HGH is a huge factor in aging, being a causative factor in osteoporosis, dementia, muscle loss, organ shrinkage, increased body-fat, skin deterioration, etc. The good news is that eating the appropriate combinations of protein, fat, and carbohydrates helps to raise HGH levels. Consistent intake of protein will raise HGH levels. Exercise, such as the programs detailed in Chapter 4 of this book will raise HGH. There are many nutritional supplements that raise HGH significantly.

THE RIGHT FOOD AT THE RIGHT TIME

*There are numerous ways to get fat—
and only one way to lose it*

There are four basic ways to get fat

1. Eat too little.
2. Eat too much.
3. Eat at the wrong times.
4. Eat the wrong combination of foods.

Numbers 1 and 4 account for 90% of the thousands of people whom I have seen over the years. It is very easy to accumulate fat. At one end of the spectrum, eating too much food causes the body to take in more calories than it can burn and stores away the extra calories in the form of body-fat. At the other end of the spectrum, depriving the body of food, activates a survival mechanism to combat starvation. This is known as the starvation protection mechanism. When food is finally ingested, even the right food, the body again stores it away as fat, in preparation for what it believes will be a starvation period.

*There is, however, only one way to lose fat:
Eat the right amount of the right food at the right time.*

After answering the "Is This You?" questions in Chapter 6, you will be directed to the plan that best suits your individual requirements. Once you find the right plan, you will discover what the right foods are, when the right times are, and what the right amounts are. You will gain the knowledge of proper food combining that is absolutely essential to your success. In combining foods appropriately, you will take control of your metabolism by taking control of your hormones. By bringing the correct balance back to your hormones, you can change your destiny.

Correct combinations of foods is the key to mastering your metabolism.

To gain a better understanding of food combining, let's first take a look at some *improper* combinations. Combinations that are certain to result in the accumulation of body-fat, and lead to a higher risk of diseases, lower energy, and an overall lack of wellness.

One great example of how one might incorrectly combine foods, and promote the storage of body-fat would be eating a piece of fruit by itself—without any protein or fats. This is a surefire way to get fat. When fruit is eaten alone, it causes the level of sugar (glucose) in your blood to rise very rapidly. The sudden surge of sugar into the bloodstream causes the release of the hormone insulin. Insulin's primary function is to remove sugar from the blood.

To remove the sugar from the blood, insulin can only do one of two things with it. It can either send the glucose into a cell to be used as energy—right now. Or second, if your cells do not need the sugar—all of it—at that very moment, insulin will store it away inside of a fat cell to be used at a later time. Because your liver converts a type of sugar found in fruit called fructose, directly into fat, the consumption of fruit alone may also elevate the amount of triglycerides (fat) in the blood.

On the other hand, had you just eaten a little bit of low-fat cheese (or any protein) with that fruit, the hormonal response would be totally different. For one, by slowing the digestion of the fruit, you would have minimized the entry of glucose into the bloodstream. In turn, this would minimize the release of insulin into the bloodstream, thus eliminating the conversion of glucose to body-fat. Also, you would cause the release of body-fat-friendly hormones, such as glucagon and HGH, which cause the body to **burn** body-fat, build muscle and bone density, and produce more energy.

Another common food-combining mistake made by many dieters is eating a bowl of cereal with nonfat milk in the morning. The highly refined carbohydrate content of the cereal and the sugars in the milk spell trouble for the well-meaning dieter. (Many people are misled into believing that milk is a high-protein food. Milk has almost twice as many carbohydrates as it has proteins.) The overload of carbohydrates causes a surge of insulin, a drop in glucagon, a rise in cortisol, and a lower level of HGH. This is absolutely the opposite of what the dieter really wants. This hormonal reaction to food creates more fat, lowers energy, makes more cravings for sugars, and raises likelihood of many diseases.

On the other hand, eating the cereal with some low-fat milk, together with a few egg whites or maybe a quick protein shake, gives much different and far better results. You see, the little bit of fat in the milk would have slowed the release of the sugars into the bloodstream, and the protein would have assisted this as well. In addition, the protein would have inhibited the release of insulin, supported the release of glucagon and HGH, and turned off the hormone cortisol.

We can optimize metabolic (hormonal) response when there is an ideal combination of protein, carbohydrate, and fat. This food combining allows the release of glucose, proteins, and fats into the bloodstream over a longer period of time, and promotes minimal insulin and cortisol secretion with maximal glucagon and HGH output.

The right food at the right time is different for each individual. That is why any one diet is only successful for a maximum of 30% of the people who try it. It is only when you determine what the right food at the right time is for *you*, that you will achieve body-fat reduction on a permanent basis, and enjoy optimum wellness.

What is the right food at the right time for you?

The right food at the right time is something that until now has been extremely difficult to figure out. What is the right food at the right time? Do you require a lot of protein? Do you require a lot of carbohydrates? Do you require a lot of fat? Do you require a lot of all of the above? How many calories should you have? How many meals should you have each day? What vitamins and minerals should you be taking? The answers to these types of questions have been very elusive—until now.

Never before has this information been available to the general public. Never before has there been one resource where you can find a nutritional program that will give you the results you desire, **no matter what your needs are**. At the beginning of the second half of this book, you will see a questionnaire chapter called, "Is This You?" By taking your time to carefully answer all of the questions in this survey, you will be directed to an ideally suited nutritional program. When you are on this nutritional program, you will discover the appropriate amounts, times, and types of foods for you. When you determine what **the right food at the right time** is for you, you will reduce body-fat in a dramatic and lasting fashion, you will feel more vital and energetic than you ever have, and you will have lasting and tangibly improved overall health.

## 3

EXERCISE

*Contrary to popular belief, exercise
is not the key to body-fat reduction*

I have helped thousands of people achieve very low levels of body-fat without their doing any exercise at all. Some are disabled and cannot exercise, and others just do not have the time or the desire to exercise. I have had clients in wheelchairs become quite lean.

I have also had hundreds of clients come in to see me for the first time complaining that no matter how much exercise they do, they just can't get any results. Does this sound familiar? I'm sure you know people who spend countless hours in the gym without significant changes in their appearance. More than 75% of all persons who exercise are not satisfied with their results. The reason for this startling statistic is that many people fall victim to the *misconception that exercise is the answer to all their troubles. It isn't.*

Even I was victimized by this misconception. Long before I studied nutrition, I was a competitive bodybuilder. In this sport, one has to achieve extremely low levels of body-fat, and a high level of muscularity. During the preparation for my first significant competition, I found myself unable to eliminate the last few pounds of body-fat. I was doing two hours of cardiovascular exercise, and one hour of weight training per day, six days a week. I just couldn't get the fat off. In fact, because of my inadequate diet, my body was unable to recover from these extreme workouts and, as a result, my body was beginning to get flabby. One day, while I was on the treadmill, one of my competitors approached me and told me he could see that I was struggling. He offered his advice. "It's your diet," he said, and recommended what I should eat. Immediately after I made the recommended changes, I began to see a whole new appearance emerge. Daily, my body became more defined, my muscles grew, and I finally achieved the physique I had been training for all that time. So you see, it was not until I changed my diet that it all came together.

This common misconception also frustrated the many of the celebrities I have helped over the years. As you know, the people on the big screen have to look their very best. That is partially why they are paid huge salaries for their work. In every celebrity case I've handled, they were already exercising when they came to me for help. Often very frustrated, many of them had live-in trainers on staff 24 hours per day. In every case, it was only when they combined all of the exercise *with proper diet* that they began to see real results.

The content of this chapter may be shocking. It may challenge everything you *think* you know about exercise. It may at times seem that I am not in favor of exercise, and am against the very notion of it. Nothing could be further from the truth. Like many of you, I am an exercise junkie. I love the sweat, the muscle burn, and the way it makes me look and feel. In fact, I am definitely an exercise advocate. I was able to pay for my Ph.D. by being a personal trainer, and have trained many other personal trainers. I would like to give you the benefit of my knowledge, research, and the thousands of hours I have spent in the gym.

What follows is not my opinion. These are hard, cold facts, which have been taken from numerous scientific studies from around the world. Let's take a look at some current statistics. In the United States alone, over $5 billion are spent each year on exercise. We have more people exercising worldwide than ever before. Here in the USA, more persons per capita are involved in an exercise routine than any other place in the world. With all these people exercising, isn't it a big surprise that more people will die this year of a heart disease than ever before? And more people dying here in the USA than elsewhere? You bet. The numbers are staggering— approximately 500,000 people, ten times the number of people an average baseball stadium can hold, will die of heart disease in the USA in 1998. More people will die of strokes and cancer this year than last. More people will die from the complications of diabetes this year than the last. High blood pressure will force many millions of *exercising* Americans to begin taking blood pressure medication this year—why? Exercise is supposed to protect us from all these maladies.

> *I'm not saying don't exercise,*
> *I'm putting the importance of*
> *exercise in perspective.*

Statistics suggest that people who vigorously exercise over long periods of time are nearly as likely to suffer a myocardial infarction (heart attack) as people who are sedentary. Numerous studies done all over the world have been inconclusive as to whether exercise can lower cholesterol. In studies where exercise has lowered cholesterol, it was not by a significant amount, and the results tended to be temporary. Exercise has not proven to have any long-term benefit to blood pressure. In any study where exercise was able to lower blood pressure, it was accomplished by means of a reduction of body-fat. When the participants of the studies went back to their old lifestyles, that is to say that they stopped exercising, their blood pressure returned to levels that were present prior to the study. Blood pressure *rises* during exercise. Exercise puts strain on the heart and circulatory system. Blood pressure can, and often does, increase to extremely high levels during weight training. If exercise is going to benefit your cardiovascular system, it will do so only when combined with proper diet. Statistics show that people who engage in exercise programs to lower their blood pressure or cholesterol fail to do so over 80% of the time.

Studies also show that exercise may actually *increase* your risk of certain cancers, especially in the absence of proper diet. This is due to the increased rate of oxidation that occurs during exercise. Oxidation is well documented to be a causative factor in cancers and other diseases. Oxidation is also well known to accelerate aging of tissues—especially skin. During exercise, oxidation can increase by up to 18,000 times the normal rate. The increase in oxidation can be counterbalanced with proper diet, again showing that diet is the key—not exercise.

If exercise were the issue, more people would be thin. If exercise were the issue, the general population would have fewer heart attacks, less cancer, fewer strokes, less hypercholesterolemia, diabetes, and cardiovascular disease. We have more people exercising than ever before, and yet all these maladies that exercise is supposed to curtail are on the rise. Surely, I'm not saying that exercise is causing all this. The point is that exercise is not preventing or curing any of it.

Exercise Is Not the Key to Reducing Body-fat. It's All in Your Diet.

However, *exercise combined with proper diet d*oes have potential benefits. If you want better muscle strength and tone, you must exercise. You can achieve a great deal of stress relief with exercise. You can achieve a significant amount of fat reduction by *combining* a properly designed and executed dietary plan with the right amount of cardiovascular and resistance exercise. You can achieve better skin tone and texture through exercise. You can reduce your level of anxiety by exercising. With a properly designed exercise program you can gain strength, stamina, and piece of mind. You may have better concentration and memory, because of more blood flow to your brain, as well as other benefits. In short, exercise must be *combined* with proper diet to have significant benefit.

The remainder of this chapter **will help you figure out what type of exercise routine will work for you**.

BASIC EXERCISE ROUTINE FOR MAXIMAL BODY-FAT REDUCTION

What follows is a basic guideline for exercise. The plan is intended for persons who are in good health. Please see your medical doctor before beginning this routine.

The exercise plan will be a combination of resistance training and cardiovascular exercise. It is imperative that you combine resistance training and cardiovascular training to achieve the greatest results. Even though you may not want to "build muscle," it is essential for you to include resistance training in your program. You see, by working your muscles with resistance, you make them more metabolically active—they will burn more calories at rest. This higher rate of calorie burning will mean faster and easier fat loss, and a much greater energy level.

THE PROGRAM

For the program to be effective, you will need to exercise between three and five days per week. If you do the cardiovascular exercise on the same days as your resistance training, it will be three. If you are going to do resistance training and cardiovascular exercise on different days, it will be five days a week. Each workout will take a minimum of 30 minutes and a maximum of 1 hour.

Keep in mind that *exercise is not mandatory*, especially in the beginning stages of your program. Because it does not cause a huge reduction of body-fat, you won't see amazing differences. However, after the fat comes off and you can see the finer details of your body, exercise will create significant changes in the shape and firmness of your muscles, which will make a startling difference in your appearance.

THE TWO MAJOR TYPES OF EXERCISE

Weight (Resistance) Training

Weight (resistance) training is an important part of your exercise program. This type of exercise tones and firms muscles, it improves the metabolism, it increases the number of calories you burn at rest, increases energy, etc.

Each muscle group will be exercised with weights (resistance) one time per week. Arms once, shoulders once, legs once, chest once, etc. Abdominal muscles will be exercised two to three times per week.

To assure your safety and the effectiveness of your workout, you should consider using a personal trainer at least once. A personal trainer will show you the proper way to do each and every exercise and help you to get things done effectively. As this is not an exercise book *per se*, I will not go into great details about how to perform various exercises. If you are unclear about any term that I use in this chapter, you should definitely consult a personal trainer. I have not used diagrams or photographs for any of the exercises specifically to prevent you from doing them improperly, limiting your results, and possibly injuring yourself.

Cardiovascular (Aerobic) Training

Cardiovascular exercise has many benefits. They include more energy, improved libido, slightly increased speed of fat reduction, better endurance, etc.

Cardiovascular (aerobic) exercise should always be done *after* the weight training portion of you workout (if you are doing both on the same day). The reason for this is simple. While you are working out with the weights, you will use most of the available sugar in your body, which will force your body to use fat for the energy required to complete the cardiovascular exercise.

To have any significant fat-burning effect, cardiovascular exercise must be done for a period of at least 40 minutes. It will make a significant difference if you extend the time to 60 minutes. Additionally, cardiovascular exercise should be performed with a precise level of intensity. The appropriate level of intensity is determined by your pulse rate. Maintaining this level of intensity insures that you will be burning the most fat possible.

When you do not follow this formula, your ability to burn fat will be at the very least, limited.

Fat-Burning Formula

220 minus your age = _____

Take that number and multiply it by 70–80%. This is the most effective heart rate and the level of intensity you should try to maintain.

Example

220 – 35 yrs. = 185. (185 × 70% = 129.) (185 × 80% = 148.)

So, if you are 35 years of age, the most effective intensity level for your cardiovascular workout will be whatever it takes to get your pulse rate to 129–148 beats per minute.

If you were walking on the treadmill and found that your pulse was 109 beats per minute, you would either increase the speed or the incline angle of the treadmill until your pulse rate went up to at least 129 beats per minute. Conversely, if your pulse rate were 160 beats per minute, you would slow the speed or reduce the incline until you saw that the pulse rate had dropped to less than 148 beats per minute.

You can take your pulse manually at the wrist by placing your index and middle fingers on the area just beneath the thumb pad on the palm of your hand. Sometimes it is difficult to find and count your pulse, especially when you are exercising. To simplify the practice of measuring your pulse rate, you can purchase an inexpensive heart rate monitor at the local sporting goods store.

SAMPLE ROUTINE

Here is an example of how you put together a muscle-toning, fat-burning workout.

Again, it is a very good idea to hire a personal trainer to teach you a specific routine for your individual needs.

- Each upper body muscle gets 2–3 sets, 12–14 repetitions per set. (Once weekly)
- Each lower body muscle gets 3–4 sets, 12–14 repetitions per set. (Once weekly)
- Women should lift a weight that is approximately 60% of the absolute maximum that they could handle for this number of repetitions. Men should be at about 75% of their maximum.
- Move from one muscle group to the other without rest. When you have worked all of the upper body muscles, take 30 seconds

of rest. With lower body muscles you will need 60 seconds of rest. This is known as a circuit. Repeat circuit 3–4 times.

- Abdominal muscles should be worked one to three times per week. Various crunching exercises are used to work the abdominal muscles. There are also different kinds of machines available for the home and also at the gym that are great for the abdominal muscles. *Do not do sit-ups.* Sit-ups are very hard on the back and not effective for the abdominal muscles either. Do four sets for the abdominal muscles, 20–40 repetitions per set. It is more important to focus on the intensity of the exercise than the number of repetitions or sets. You should achieve a significant "burn" in the abdominal muscles on each set. You should *not* feel pain anywhere else, especially not in your neck or back. You don't have to lift "weights." There are stretchable rubber tubes you can use, many different kinds of machines available, etc., that will provide the same effect. You can even use plastic bags filled with sand or water as weights.

- *After* each of your resistance training workouts, you should stretch. Stretching is always *done at the end of the workout* because this is when you want to elongate and relax the muscles. It makes absolutely no sense to relax a muscle that you are about to tense and flex. (Bear in mind that the #1 cause of exercise-related injury is overflexibility.) Stretching is an important part of working out that is very often neglected.

Stretching is important for many reasons. Stretching makes the muscles look better. It keeps your body flexible and reduces chance of muscle pulls. It improves circulation. It increases endurance. There are many additional reasons to stretch—so do not neglect it. Each workout, stretch the muscles that were worked that day, as well as your lower back and abdominal area. By frequently stretching these areas, you will reduce the chance of an injury to your lower back by about 80%. Remember not to "bounce" when you stretch. Use slow, deliberate movements and hold each fully stretched position for at least thirty seconds.

Once again, this is a basic routine, one that will be universally acceptable. You can make changes based on your goals, handicaps, time restraints, etc. Remember that exercise is not going to make you or break you. It is merely an accessory to the main component of your program—your diet.

## 4

OPTIMAL DIGESTION

> *WARNING:*
> *Digestive problems will severely*
> *inhibit your body's ability to burn fat!*
> *Proper digestion is an absolutely critical*
> *factor in fat reduction*

Because the digestive/gastrointestinal system performs over a hundred different duties, in addition to digesting food and nutrients, it is arguably the most important system in the body. It is essential that this system be working at its fullest capacity for you to enjoy maximum results from any of the 10 nutritional plans in this book.

Any food, vitamin, mineral, antioxidant, or other nutrient must be properly processed by the gastrointestinal (GI) tract in order for your body to extract its full benefit. In fact, many types of foods and nutrients will actually do harm to your body if they are not processed correctly. As an example, it is important to get enough of the mineral calcium. If you are taking extra calcium that your body is unable to process correctly, it can lead to various problems in the body, which include kidney stones and calcium deposits. Proteins that are not fully digested will putrefy (rot) in the intestines, causing gas, pain, bloating, and a toxic bowel.

It is imperative that this system be working correctly as you begin the appropriate diet plan. If you are suffering from gas, bloating, heartburn, diarrhea, stomach/intestinal pain—cramps, ulcers, belching after meals, excessive fullness after normal size meals, constipation, or bubbles/gurgles in the stomach, you *must* read this chapter before beginning your diet.

THE GI TRACT NEVER SLEEPS

The gastrointestinal (GI) tract is a totally automatic and very efficient machine. It is working 24 hours per day, whether you've eaten or not. It requires no conscious thought, and performs many functions other than just digestion of the food we eat. Because the digestive system functions automatically, people give it very little thought—until it doesn't work any more. Then the gas, bloating, cramping, heartburn, belching, and pain demand attention. Usually that attention is in the form of a medication, one that will make the symptoms go away. After the symptoms have been relieved, the person once again forgets about the GI tract, until another episode takes place and the person is forced again to take medication. Sooner or later, this pattern develops into a chronic situation, and persons find themselves consuming various symptom-relieving medications on a permanent daily schedule.

Unfortunate persons who find themselves with "tummy trouble," need to ask two important questions: why does my stomach hurt? and how can I fix whatever has gone wrong?

Instead, many will turn to either an over-the-counter medication, or they will be prescribed a medication by a well-meaning doctor who wants them to feel better. In very few cases will the cause of the problem be searched for. This is regrettable. The cause of the problem is often very simple to uncover, and once it has been found, the person can enjoy lasting relief without continually taking medication. (Medication that may have serious side effects.)

DIGESTIVE PROBLEMS ARE AT THE HEART OF MANY ILLNESSES

Digestive dysfunction is among the most widespread afflictions in America today. The numbers are overwhelming. It is estimated that over **70% of all Americans have digestive disorders.**

Can you fathom the enormity of this problem? **Half of all adults** and ⅕ **of all children** are suffering some form of gastrointestinal disorder. Digestive and GI problems are within the top two most common reasons for visits to medical doctors, *second only to the common cold.* According to the US Department of Health and Human Services, digestive illness has *cost U.S. taxpayers $50 billion each year,* and has resulted in approximately 270 million days of lost time in sick days, which is an additional $15–20 billion per year!

Of course, this monumental problem hasn't gone unnoticed by the pharmaceutical companies. Digestive dysfunction has become big business. Zantac, a medication most often prescribed for indigestion and heartburn, is the #1 drug sold today, with annual sales reaching over $1 billion. Clearly, this problem has exceeded epidemic proportions, and the problem is only getting worse each year.

In reading this book, you may be hearing this information for the first time. Because digestive dysfunction is so far-reaching, and because so many of my patients' problems revolve around this issue, and because it affects the overall well-being of so many millions of people, *this issue must be given top priority.* In particular, this critical matter is one of the primary reasons that I wrote this book. Millions of people in the United States are sick, many more millions worldwide—sick with illnesses that can be easily treated and prevented by giving attention to these internal issues. People could feel so much better—so quickly—that I felt passionately that a public forum for this information *had* to be established. In fact, I'm assuming that you could very well be the person that I intended to reach with this information.

Digestive and gastrointestinal problems are at the very core of many of our nation's major illnesses. These illnesses use up a large part of our nation's healthcare budget. You can clearly see that digestive problems are part of a very large picture.

When your body is not able to process food and nutrients properly, nutrient deficiencies occur, and these nutrient deficiencies can, and often do result in a very wide array of illnesses.

Gastrointestinal problems and digestive inadequacy are directly or indirectly linked to all of the following conditions: arthritis, auto-immune diseases, eczema, food sensitivities, migraine headaches, constipation, chronic fatigue, abdominal pain, forms of asthma, joint pain, muscle pain, confusion, mood swings, nervousness, poor exercise tolerance, poor immune system function, recurrent vaginal yeast infections, skin rashes, psoriasis, bladder infections, fevers, poor memory, shortness of breath, bloating, nausea, diarrhea, gurgling in the stomach, cramping, liver toxicity, heartburn, bloating, Addison's disease, lupus, myasthenia gravis, celiac disease, osteoporosis, dermatitis, herpes, pernicious anemia, diabetes, gall bladder disease, acne rosacia, Grave's disease, Sjogrens's syndrome, viral toxicosis, hepatitis, hyper- and hypothyroidism, chronic hives, vitaligo, iron deficiency, parasitic infection, and attention deficit disorder.

These conditions and many others can all be caused and/or exacerbated by digestive problems. To determine whether you may have digestive dysfunction, please fill out the following questionnaire. I have administered this test to thousands of my patients and I have found it to be very effective in determining whether there is any need for concern.

Table 04.01

Digestive Screening

Please answer the following questions using this scale:

- 0 = less than once per month
- 1 = more than once per month
- 2 = once per week
- 3 = three times per week
- 4 = daily

Do you feel nauseous? _____

Do you have gas? _____

Do you have abdominal bloating? _____

Do you get gassy/bloated after meals? _____

Do you get reflux or heartburn? _____

Do you have less than one bowel
movement per day? _____

Are your stools compact and hard to pass? _____

Do you have diarrhea? _____

Do you have gurgles in your stomach? _____

Do you belch following meals? _____

Do you travel outside the U.S.? _____

Have you had an ulcer? Yes = 4 _____

Do you have abdominal/intestinal pain? _____

TOTAL _____

SCORING YOUR QUESTIONNAIRE

If you scored 0–6 on the questionnaire, there is minimal concern that you have or are suffering from any form of digestive dysfunction. If you scored 7–12, it is likely that you have digestive dysfunction, and should continue reading. If you scored 13–17, it is highly likely that you have digestive dysfunction. If you scored 18 or higher, you absolutely positively have digestive dysfunction. Learning how you can remedy this situation will save you from suffering any longer, and in extreme cases, may even save your life.

IF YOU HAVE SCORED 12 OR MORE, IT IS IMPERATIVE THAT YOU READ ON

If you have scored above 12 on this questionnaire, I would highly recommend that you undergo a simple laboratory test. This test can be taken in the privacy of your own home, and involves collecting a small stool sample, and sending it into the lab for testing. This simple procedure will detect the *causes* of many different kinds of gastrointestinal/digestive problems. From this very specific and highly specialized test, we can uncover the hidden causes of many illnesses, and create a solution for your specific problem. The test will indicate levels of unhealthful bacteria, the presence of parasites, and levels of digestive enzymes, presence of inflammation, intolerance of certain foods, levels of yeast in the GI tract, and other facts about your digestive system. By remedying this issue now, you will significantly increase the amount of fat you will burn on *any* of the ten diets in this book. In addition, you will get significant relief from pain and suffering, you may prevent serious disease, and you will feel better than you ever have. Once these problems are corrected, they are corrected forever *unless you return to your "old ways."*

If you are suffering from a digestive/ gastrointestinal problem, remedy the situation now. It may save your life. It will definitely improve your results.

If you have scored 12 or higher on the digestive screening, and would like to put an end to your suffering by having the test performed, you may call toll free (888) 663–2881, to order a test kit. When the results of your test are in, they will be reviewed with you, and recommendations will be made as to how you will correct the problems. The methods of correcting these problems are usually very simple and these corrections can be made in a short amount of time. It is extremely rare that one would require any medications or surgeries. In 99% of all cases, simple nutritional supplements are all that is necessary, and then it usually takes only a few weeks to achieve total elimination of the problems. You can also start on your food plan while taking care of these problems.

You may also choose to call the laboratory directly. This laboratory can provide you with the name and telephone number of a trained physician in your area who can order these specialized tests, interpret the results, and recommend a treatment.

Diagnos-Techs Laboratory: (800) 878–3787

You may also choose to use your own physician, but if the correct test is not ordered from this specific laboratory, the information will not be useful, and in the end, will be of no benefit to you. In medicine there is a saying: "Doctors are only as good as their data."

As I stated in the opening sentence of this chapter, the digestive/gastrointestinal system is very complex. To gain an understanding of how your digestive tract works and what can happen when it does not work correctly, take a few moments to read the rest of this chapter.

HOW THE DIGESTIVE SYSTEM WORKS— A GUIDED TOUR THROUGH THE GASTROINTESTINAL TRACT

The digestive tract is like a hose that runs from one end of your body to the other. This hose ranges from 20 to 30 feet in length. The surface area of this hose is often larger than the surface of a tennis court. Its function is to turn the food and various types of nutrients that you eat into microscopic particles that the cells can use for energy, growth, and repair. The old saying, "You are what you eat" is definitely *not* true. The saying should be, *"You are what happens to what you eat."* Certainly, nutritious foods are the right place to start on the path to leanness and wellness, but many people eat the right foods and still have problems. Many of you are following a very appropriate diet right now, but because your digestive tract does not process what you eat correctly, you are not able to benefit from that food. Adequate digestion is the very first step in obtaining optimal wellness and top physical shape. Even more important than what you eat, is what your body does with what you eat.

Chewing thoroughly is the first step of optimal digestion.

It all begins with the mouth, where the food is chewed and liquefied. The first step of digestion occurs when you are chewing. Saliva softens food, and enzymes contained within the saliva begin to digest carbohydrates. As the food is swallowed, it is passed through the esophagus, the tube that leads from your mouth to your stomach. In a process called peristalsis, the food is pushed through the espophagial tract. In six to ten seconds the food reaches a door called the esophageal sphincter, which opens to allow the food into the stomach. The esophageal sphincter keeps ingested food and acids within the stomach, and prevents their traveling upwards. In some cases, the esophageal sphincter does not close properly, and this results in a condition known as "acid reflux." In this condition, feelings of warmth, burning, and pressure in the chest and throat, result from contents of the stomach traveling back up into these areas. In many cases, the "reflux" is actually caused by bile, which is not acidic at all. The bile is alkaline, or the opposite of acidic, and yet it can cause a significant burning sensation.

The Stomach

After the food has traveled down through the esophagus, it enters the stomach. The stomach is located just under the rib cage, just underneath the heart. The stomach's main function is to secrete hydrochloric acid into the food sitting inside it. Hydrochloric acid is a very potent acid that begins to break down the proteins, minerals, and fats, and also to destroy the majority of bacteria that are in our everyday foods. Stomach (hydrochloric) acid also activates enzymes that are contained in the foods we eat, and those produced by our bodies. After the food has been in the stomach for a period ranging from 4–20 minutes, it will be transported by gravity and peristalsis into the small intestine.

The Small Intestine

The small intestine is hardly small. When measured in length, it can be as long as 20 feet. Cut open and spread flat, it would cover the surface area of an average home. The small intestine is where the food and nutrients are completely digested. Nutrients, vitamins, and minerals are absorbed through the wall of the small intestine, which acts very much like a filter. This filter blocks out the toxins, fiber, and bacteria and lets the proteins, fats, carbohydrates, and nutrients into the bloodstream. Certain medications can damage the intestinal surface, rendering it unable to perform its tasks. Certain medications will cause inflammation of the intestine, thus blocking out passage of certain nutrients, while other drugs will increase the size of the microscopic holes in the intestine that allow the very tiny particles of food to pass through into the blood. This is known as increased intestinal permeability. Increased permeability of the intestine can result in a wide array of illnesses, including arthritis, asthma, psoriasis, and autoimmune disorders.

The small intestine has three basic segments: the duodenum, the jejunum, and the ileum. The duodenum makes up the first foot or so. The jejunum makes up 35–45% percent of the total length of the small intestine, and the ileum comprises the final segment of the small intestine.

After the food reaches the first section of the small intestine, the duodenum, it encounters digestive enzymes that have been secreted by the pancreas.

The Pancreas

The pancreas is an organ that lies directly in the middle of the torso, right against the rear of the abdominal cavity. The pancreas has two main functions: the production of digestive enzymes, and the production of the hormone insulin. It is critically important to the body for the pancreas to produce all of the enzymes necessary for the digestion of food. Pancreatic insufficiency, which describes a condition in which the pancreas does not produce enough of the necessary enzymes, is becoming more common. When an inadequate amount of enzymes are present, the food that is consumed will not be fully digested before traveling further down the intestinal tract. When this happens, the undigested food begins to ferment and putrefy within the intestines, and this causes gas, bloating, burping, discomfort and indigestion. This condition is easily corrected. The test, mentioned earlier in this chapter, can give the information needed to bring the pancreas back to health. Usually all that is required to revive the pancreas is supplementation with digestive enzymes, in pill or liquid form, taken at mealtime.

Once the necessary enzymes have completely digested the food down into microscopically small particles, and that food is moving through the duodenum, on its way into the ileum, it is met by a flow of bile. Bile is secreted by the gall bladder.

The Gall Bladder

The gall bladder is a pear-shaped organ that rests just below the liver, on the lower right side of the front of the torso. Its main function is to concentrate and store bile. Bile emulsifies, softens and liquefies fats and cholesterol and fat-soluble vitamins by breaking them down into very small globules. This creates a bigger surface area for fat-splitting enzymes to attach to, and thereby increasing the enzymes' efficiency in digesting these molecules. Bile also takes the highly acidic food mixture and turns it into a more alkaline mixture, thus protecting the intestines from damage by the acid. In between meals, the gall bladder stores bile to use the next time we eat. The gall bladder can become dysfunctional, producing too little, or too much bile. In addition, stones can form in the gall bladder, resulting in a very painful condition that often leads to the surgical removal of the organ. In my opinion, 90% of all gall bladder removals may be unnecessary. In many cases, the gall bladder has become dysfunctional as a result of long-term poor diet, use of certain medications, inadequate secretion of pancreatic enzymes, and stress. Regaining proper dietary intake, improving the pancreatic function, discontinuing the offending medication, and lowering stress levels will bring the gall bladder back to health.

The Colon

As the food continues its journey through the intestinal tract, passing through the jejunum and ileum, it reaches its final destination—the large intestine. Once the majority of nutrients have been absorbed, the water, toxins, bacteria, and the fiber pass through what is called ileocecal valve and into the large intestine or what we call the colon. The ileocecal valve is just near your right hipbone and separates the contents of the small and large intestine. The colon is short—only 3 to 5 feet long—and its purpose is to absorb water and the remaining nutrients from the bowel material and to form stool. About 2½ gallons of water pass through the large intestine every day, ⅔ of which is derived from your own body fluids. The efficient colon pulls 80% of the water out of the material, which is absorbed into the bloodstream. The large intestine or colon has three main parts: the ascending, which is up the right side of the body; the transverse, which goes straight behind the belly button; and the descending, which travels downward on the left side of the body and ends at the rectum. Stool exits from the rectum.

Beneficial Bacteria

Stool begins to form and solidify in the transverse part of the colon. Astoundingly, ⅓ of a healthy person's stool material is comprised of *bacteria!* Many trillions of bacteria are passed from the healthy colon on a daily basis. Four or five hundred different types of bacteria are usually present in your digestive system, each of which have different types and strains. The colon contains trillions and trillions of bacteria, growing and multiplying on a minute-to-minute basis. Bacteria are capable of reproducing very quickly, often in less than a second. As new bacteria are born within the GI tract, overcrowding occurs, causing the old bacteria to be pushed out with the stool as it exits the body. The large majority of the bacteria within the GI tract are beneficial, indeed *essential*, to the human body. You may have heard of these bacteria. One is lactobacillus acidophilus. Another is bifodobacterium. Believe it or not, there is even a form of the feared E.Coli that is a welcome tenant within the GI tract. These essential bacteria play many different roles in the body. They help us fight infections. They boost our immune systems. They increase the body's ability to metabolize vitamins and minerals. They increase our resistance to food poisoning. They help us to digest food. They help regulate the muscles within the intestinal tract. They produce antibiotics and anti-fungal substances, which help prevent other unhealthful organisms from living within the intestinal tract. They help us to produce beneficial forms of fat within the body. They produce anti-toxins. They help prevent tumors and have anti-cancer effects. They protect us from heavy metals. They help keep triglycerides and cholesterol under control. They help to break down and rebuild hormones, and they also promote a healthy metabolism. These beneficial bacteria are absolutely critical to our wellness and longevity.

One of the most common problems of the digestive tract is the *elimination of the essential intestinal bacteria*. Six out of 10 people have either totally eliminated the "good" bacteria from their bodies, or have reduced them to alarmingly low levels. When this happens, all of the functions of the digestive tract will deteriorate over time. In addition to digestive problems, the absence of these essential inhabitants contribute to a multitude of other problems, ranging from PMS to cancer.

The elimination of the essential intestinal bacteria is caused by a number of different things. For example, one strong course of antibiotics will eliminate every last one of the trillions and trillions of beneficial bacteria in the body. The antibiotic was taken for that very reason—to eliminate bacteria. The problem is, of course, that these drugs are not selective. They are on a mission to eliminate any and all bacteria. Now I'm not saying that you should never take antibiotics, just that you should not take them unless absolutely necessary, and if you do take them, take a supplemental form of the good bacteria after you are done with the cycle of antibiotics. These bacteria can be purchased from health food stores and come in powder, pills, and liquid. I must warn you, though, that these bacteria are very sensitive to heat, light, air, and contaminants. It is very common to find products on the shelves of health food stores that do not contain *any living bacteria*. You should make certain that these bacteria, or for that matter, any supplement, come from a reliable and responsible manufacturer. If you should have any questions about where you can obtain supplementation, you may call toll-free (888) 663–2881.

Another common way that the beneficial bacteria are destroyed is by the consumption of chlorinated tap water. The chlorine was added to the water to kill bacteria. When the chlorine reaches the intestine, it kills the bacteria as well. Especially the beneficial ones, as they are so sensitive. I recommend you find a source of water that is not chlorinated. Once again, if you have been drinking a significant amount of chlorinated water, you should consider replenishing your body's supply of beneficial intestinal bacteria.

Common food preservatives can also decrease the numbers of beneficial bacteria. These additives are used in our food supplies to eliminate any bacteria from the food. Once ingested, these substances do what they were invented to do—kill bacteria. Consumption of alcohol can also harm our intestinal bacteria. A small amount of alcohol is not a major concern; however, a six-pack here and there is a problem.

These beneficial bacteria do not just appear magically. You cannot get any significant amount from any type of food, milk, etc. You must purposefully put them back into your body after they are gone, or suffer the consequences. The beneficial intestinal bacteria are populated into the GI tract of a fetus while in the womb. After birth, the breastfeeding baby will be fed the good bacteria, which is contained in breastmilk. Babies who are not breastfed will begin life with reduced numbers of the good bacteria, which will affect nearly every area of the child's development.

A FINAL WORD FOR THOSE WHO
HAVE "TUMMY TROUBLE"

After reading this chapter, I'm sure you have a new understanding about your GI tract and the monumental importance of its proper function. You have learned that any type of eating plan will not be effective unless you are able to process the food. Now, I'm sure that you are probably very excited to begin your diet, but you really should take a moment to investigate why you have gas, bloating, heartburn, and other discomforts. You will reap the rewards in a big way.

On the other hand, if you disregard the information from this chapter and begin a food plan without getting a clear picture of what is happening within your body, you will be disappointed with the results—*I promise.*

## 5

NUTRITIONAL SUPPLEMENTS THAT MAY ACCELERATE BODY-FAT REDUCTION

Always remember that nutritional supplements can be truly effective only when combined with the right diet

NUTRITIONAL SUPPLEMENTS CAN ENHANCE THE RATE OF YOUR BODY-FAT LOSS UP TO 30%

Nutritional supplements can be a very helpful ally on the war against body-fat. In addition to the appropriate nutritional program, you may choose to take some natural and effective supplementation to get the best return for your efforts. Simply following the appropriate nutritional program guarantees that you will experience significant results. In some cases, however, additional nutritional supplementation can extend those fantastic results by as much as 30%.

I have compiled reams of data on these supplements, and have created a list of the finest, safest, and most revolutionary supplements available. Most of us have seen news reports about harmful and dangerous effects caused by drugs that have been pushed on the public for weight loss. It is always amazing to me that some would jeopardize their long-term health (and in some dramatic cases, their life) for a promise to "get thin quick." Please remember, there is no such thing. If you have 100 pounds of fat to lose, diet drugs, stomach stapling, and starvation are not the healthy way to go about it. It will take some time, it may take some discipline, but you can have lasting results only by following a nutritional program that fits your particular needs.

I cannot emphasize this enough: no amount of exercise, no surgery, no weight loss drug, and no nutritional supplement will eradicate body-fat by itself. You can only burn fat by utilizing the proper nutritional program for you.

Section 1

MULTIVITAMINS/MINERALS/ANTIOXIDANTS

The most important nutritional supplement in any case is a multivitamin-mineral-antioxidant. Any single nutrient deficiency has the potential to change the way your body will respond to any diet.

Why Take a Multivitamin/Mineral/Antioxidant?

Because of soil nutrient depletion, low air quality, increased personal stress, the increasing amounts of oxidizing substances in our food supply, declining quality of foods, increased physical activity, water additives, dieting, aging, use of chemistry-altering medications and more, *it is nearly impossible to derive all of the nutri-*

ents you require from food alone. For example, just one hour in a smoke-filled room can deplete your body of an entire day's supply of vitamin C. In many cases, the very metabolic imbalances that made you need this book were caused by nutrient deficiencies.

It is absolutely essential that you maintain adequate nutrient intake while on any of the ten diet plans within this book. Your failure to do so will at least significantly hinder your progress.

This multivitamin/mineral/antioxidant formula I have developed is safe and effective for the majority of persons over 15 years of age. To obtain any of the supplements in this chapter, simply visit your local vitamin store, or you may place an order by calling toll-free (888) 663–2881.

Table 05.01

Dr. Perrone's Vitamin/Mineral/Antioxidant Formula

Each daily serving of two packets provides the following.

Vitamins and Minerals

Vitamin A (acetate)–5,000 IU

Mixed carotenoids–15,000 IU

Vitamin D (ergocalciferol)–400 IU

Vitamin E (Mixed toco-
pherols)–600 IU

Vitamin K (Phytonadione)–
100 MCG

Vitamin C (Mixed ascor-
bates)–2,500 MG

Vitamin B-1 (Thiamin HCI)–
125 MG

Vitamin B-2 (Riboflavin)–75 MG

Vitamin B-3 (Niacinamide)–
200 MG

Vitamin B-5 (Calcium pantothen-
ate)–500 MG

Vitamin B-6 (Pyridoxine
HCI)–100 MG

Vitamin B-12
(Cyanocobalamin)–200 MCG

Biotin–350 MCG

Folic acid–800 MCG

Choline (Bitartrate)–175 MG

Inositol–100 MG

Calcium (Citrate)–700 MG

Copper (Amino acid chelate)–
2 MG

Chromium (Picolinate)–400 MCG

Boron (Citrate)–2 MG

Iodine (kelp)–200 MCG

Magnesium
(Citrate/Glycinate)–500 MG

Manganese (Amino acid
chelate)–25 MG

Molybdenum (Amino acid
chelate)–125 MCG

Selenium (Selenomethionine)–
200 MCG

Potassium (Citrate)–99 MG

Para aminobenzoic acid
(PABA)–75 MG

Vanadyl sulfate–1 MG

Zinc (Amino acid chelate)–
30 MG

Additional nutrients, Antioxidants, etc.

Bilberry–100 MG

Coenzyme Q10–50 MG

Bioflavinoids–250 MG

Garlic–500 MG 4,000 MCG
Allicin

Gingko Biloba Stdzd– 60 MG

Pycnogenol–50 MG

Green tea extract–150 MG

Alpha lipoic acid–75 MG

Glutathione®–25 MG

Silymarin–50 MG

N-acetyl-cysteine–250 MG

Betaine–150 MG

Note: While the preceding formula will be effective for most, it is also a good idea to consult with your physician or a nutritionist to make sure all of your needs are being met.

Section 2

NUTRIENTS THAT MAY
ACCELERATE FAT LOSS

The following is a list of nutritional supplements that may accelerate the speed at which fat can be eliminated from your body. Although these supplements are effective, none can be even a fraction as effective as the proper diet. Never rely on supplements alone. Diet is the hub of the wheel—the foundation on which the house stands. Once you do have the right diet, and follow it consistently, only then will supplements create big differences in the rate of your fat loss.

Take a few moments to review this list and consider using one or more of these supplements. If you have any illnesses or diseases, or you are taking prescription medication, consult with your physician, or nutritionist, prior to taking these or any nutritional supplements.

L-Carnitine

This amino acid may increase the amount of fat you can burn during a cardiovascular workout. L-Carnitine is the substance your body uses to transport a fat cell across a cell wall into the mitochondria, the center of the cell, where the fat can be burned for energy. L-Carnitine supplementation may increase the amount of fat that is available to the mitochondria, which, in theory, would decrease the amount of sugar burned during exercise. Many studies have been done to determine the effectiveness of L-Carnitine for fat burning. Some have proven it to work and others have proven that it does not. My personal experience with L-Carnitine, after using it myself and with hundreds of clients, is that when used correctly, it works.

Dose: 3,000–5,000 mg. 40 minutes prior to cardiovascular exercise.

Citrimax

Citrimax products contain an herbal extract called HCA. HCA, or hydroxycitric acid, can make a big difference in the speed at which you can burn fat. HCA works in several ways. HCA inhibits an enzyme called ATP citrate lyase, and in doing so HCA decreases appetite, reduces the body's ability to make fat, and increases the body's ability to store glycogen. In my experience, using Citrimax makes a noticeable difference in the rate of fat reduction by those who use it. Citrimax may also lower cholesterol.

Dose: 2,000 mg. 30 minutes before meals.

Conjugated Linoleic Acid (CLA)

CLA is actually a very special type of fat. Recent research has shown the American diet to be deficient in this type of fat. This special fat has the ability to accelerate fat reduction in dieters and enhance muscle growth in bodybuilders. CLA may accelerate fat reduction by inhibiting an enzyme called lipoprotein lipase. This enzyme is involved in the storage of fat into fat cells. Studies that have been done using CLA with humans have had promising results. In my practice I have seen pronounced results almost every time I have recommended it. CLA can accelerate the loss of fat by up to 20%.

Dose: 3500 mg. (providing 1800 mg. CLA ea.) 5 times per day.

Chromium Picolinate or Polynicotinate

Chromium picolinate is a mineral that can make your dieting process much easier. Chromium has been shown in many studies to *cause increases in the speed of fat reduction*, help control appetite, improve the way the body metabolizes sugars and carbohydrates, and also speed up muscle growth. When used correctly, chromium picolinate will help to reduce sugar cravings too. This is one of the most widely used nutritional supplements in the world, and with good reason. Most people who use chromium report beneficial results that they can see and feel. Typically those results are lessened sugar cravings and better energy levels, along with accelerated fat reduction.

Dose: 200 mcg. 3 to 6 times per day.

Fiber supplements

Fiber supplements will benefit you in many ways. Fiber can slow down the digestion of food, causing the sugars, proteins and fats to enter the bloodstream over a longer period of time. This will reduce appetite, reduce cravings, and improve the steadiness of energy levels. Fiber keeps the intestines, especially the colon healthy. Fiber helps to feed the beneficial bacteria of the intestinal tract, which will keep digestion at its best, improve the immune system, help to balance hormones, and also help to detoxify the body. I recommend fiber supplements in almost every case.

Dose: 2–5 grams of soluble/insoluble (mix) 3–5 times per day.

Growth hormone releasing agents

There are quite a few supplements available these days that have the capability of causing the body to release extra human growth hormone. (See Chapter 2 about this hormone.) Since HGH helps to burn fat and build muscle while improving bone density and strengthening the immune system, it would definitely be in your best interest to coax your body into producing more of this substance. Many doctors even recommend injecting the hormone. Some of the more effective substances used to cause release of this hormone are: arginine, ornithine, glutamine, glycine, gaba, okg.

Dose: Varies. Please consult with a nutritionist.

Gymneme Sylvestre

This Ayurvedic Indian medicinal herb holds significant promise for the dieter who has "tried everything." Also promising for diabetics, gymneme sylvestre has, in numerous studies, been shown to be able to repair damage to the beta cells in the pancreas—where the hormone insulin is produced. Gymeneme sylvestre has also shown that it can reduce the amount of sugar in the blood, which would increase the amount of fat used for energy. This herb has the added ability of increasing the sensitivity to insulin at the cellular level, which over time, will make it much easier to reduce the fat in your body. These are significant benefits to dieters, and I certainly recommend your taking gymeneme sylvestre if you have or are prone to diabetes, or if you have tried many diets only to be frustrated by a lack of results.

Dose: 250–500 mg. (24% gymnemic acid) 30 minutes before meals.

Gugulipid

This Ayurvedic Indian herb has shown in several studies to raise the amount of circulating thyroid hormones. This would, in theory, be of benefit to the dieter or anyone with a history of thyroid trouble, or those with a family history of thyroid trouble. This herb is also very effective for lowering cholesterol and triglycerides while *raising* HDL (good) cholesterol. This supplement should be taken for 60 days, after which time you should take 14 days off. Repeat cycle as many times as desired.

Dose: 500–1000 mg. (3% gugulsterones) 4 times per day.

Ma Huang–containing products

Ma Huang is an herb with huge promise for dieters. Ma Huang has been shown to possess the ability to increase the rate of fat loss. Ma Huang has recently received much "bad press," because it has potential side effects and potential for abuse as well.

However, when used appropriately and in combination with the necessary companion herbs, Ma Huang is not only safe, but also very effective. Ma Huang *must be combined with other herbs* to promote fat loss. Those other herbs are Gotu Kola (or Kola Nut) and White Willow.

Do not use this herbal combination without first consulting with a doctor.

Dose: Check label of product.

Pyruvate

Pyruvate is a substance that has been heavily studied for its benefit to athletes and dieters. Pyruvate has the ability to increase endurance and accelerate fat loss. Nearly 100 studies have been done on Pyruvate and nearly all of them have reached similar conclusions—Pyruvate boosts endurance and speeds fat loss.

Dose: 15–30 grams per day divided between 4 doses.

Vanadyl Sulfate

Vanadyl sulfate is a specially processed form of the mineral vanadium. This exciting mineral has the ability to lower insulin levels, increase insulin sensitivity, transport glucose and protein into cells, and increase glycogen storage. Vanadyl sulfate holds promise for diabetics, as it can lower the need for exogenous insulin treatment. For the dieter, the insulin lowering effects of Vanadyl means faster fat loss, more energy, fewer cravings and stronger muscles. This supplement should be taken for no more than 90 days. After 90 days, take 30 days off. Repeat this cycle as needed, or until body-fat goals are reached.

Dose: 3 to 10 mg. taken 15–30 minutes before meals.

Yohimbe/Yohimbine

Yohimbe is very effective in helping to eliminate fat from the most stubborn of all areas, such as the hips, thighs, and abdominal areas. Yohimbe affects the Alpha 2 receptor, which is the pushbutton on a fat cell that makes it open up and store fat. Yohimbe is also a well-known aphrodisiac. Yohimbe should be taken for only 45 days at a time, after which you must take 21 days off before resuming use.

Consult with your doctor before taking Yohimbe.

Dose: 5–15 mg. of Yohimbine, 1–3 times per day.

## 6

IS THIS YOU?

Here is where the fun starts

Often those who read diet books skip over the text of the book and turn to the pages on the diet. If you have done this, please stop now, and read the information in Chapters 1–5. The information contained within those pages will greatly assist you on your journey to reduce body-fat, achieve wellness, and experience complete metabolic transformation.

What follows is a lengthy list of important questions that will guide you to the appropriate plan. Take your time and answer every question. Then take a look at your answers for each section and determine where you scored the highest. The group of questions with the highest percentage of "yes" answers will be the most effective plan for you. You may find that you scored high on more than one group of questions. If that happens, use the guidelines that appear at the beginning of each of those diet chapters to assist you in determining the best plan for you.

Take your time.

Think about the questions.

Table 06.01

Questions for the 3+2 Plan

1. You sometimes will go through most of a day without eating
2. You will be satisfied with a piece of cheese and bread
3. You have a very busy schedule, often with not even enough time to eat lunch
4. You have been on less than three diets in your life
5. Your energy could be better, but it could also be worse
6. You seem to get mid-morning slumps in your energy, even sleepiness
7. You probably won't have much time for exercise in the next few months
8. You fall asleep easily and sleep soundly
9. You are not excessively thirsty
10. You have a small amount of water retention
11. You have cravings for sweets somewhat often
12. At times, you will feel hungry, but nothing sounds good to eat
13. You have lost some weight in the past, but not many inches, and it all came back
14. You have ringing in the ears
15. You have no more than fifty pounds of fat to lose
16. Your lifestyle is high paced and sometimes hectic
17. You have a high stress job with long hours
18. You get headaches
19. You fall asleep quickly at night
20. You tap your foot or wiggle your leg

# of yes answers = ___9___ out of 20

% of yes answers ___45%___

1=5% 2=10% 3=15% 4=20% 5=25% 6=30% 7=35% 8=40%
9=45% 10=50% 11=55% 12=60% 13=65% 14=70% 15=75%
16=80% 17=85% 18=90% 19=95% 20=100%

Table 06.02

Questions for the EFA Plan

1. You have been on a lowfat or "fat-free" diet for 6 of the last 12 months
2. You have cardiovascular disease, or it runs in the family
3. You have eczema or psoriasis
4. You are frequently thirsty, even after a glass of water
5. You are losing hair at an accelerated rate
6. You have arthritis or other joint problems
7. Your wounds are slow to heal
8. Your immune system is weak
9. You have tingling in the arms and/or legs
10. You crave sweets, even after a full meal
11. You have high cholesterol
12. You have high triglycerides
13. You have dry skin
14. You cannot eat a piece of bread, you must have more if you have any
15. You feel weak and tired most of the time
16. You have diabetes
17. You have problems with vision
18. You have edema (swelling of the extremities)
19. Carbohydrate (sugar) cravings prevent you from following a diet
20. You have behavioral problems or mood disorders
21. (females) You have miscarried
22. (males) You have low sperm count
23. You sweat excessively
24. (females) You have PMS before your menstrual cycle
25. You have had liver problems

# of yes answers = ____4____ out of 25

% of yes answers ____16²____

1=4% 2=8% 3=12% 4=16% 5=20% 6=24% 7=28% 8=32%
9=36% 10=40% 11=44% 12=48% 13=52% 14=56% 15=60%
16=64% 17=68% 18=72% 19=76% 20=80% 21=84% 22=88%
23=92% 24=96% 25=100%

Table 06.03

Questions for the Protein Plus One Plan

1. You often have a mid-afternoon energy slump
2. You get sleepy after eating a meal with a large portion of carbohydrates
3. You may go many hours between meals without getting hungry
4. You feel you have low energy level most of the time
5. You need at least 8 hours of sleep
6. You crave carbohydrates
7. You desire a rapid loss of body-fat
8. You have tried dieting in the past without long-term success
9. You have at least one bowel movement per day
10. You have difficulty concentrating
11. You often feel depressed, but rarely have anxiety
12. You have difficulty in maintaining or losing weight
13. You have one or more people in my family with diabetes
14. Your hair is thinning, beyond what is reasonable to expect for a person your age
15. You have between 10 and 150 pounds to lose
16. You often urinate less than four times per day
17. When you work out, your results are not equaled by your effort
18. You have very little endurance
19. Given the opportunity to eat anything you want, proteins would be your last choice
20. You often have water retention
21. You are at least 14 years of age
22. You often crave salty foods
23. You often get more than three colds or flus per year
24. You have little desire to eat breakfast first thing in the morning
25. You have difficulty following a highly structured dietary plan

# of yes answers = ___14___ out of 25

% of yes answers ___56%___

1=4% 2=8% 3=12% 4=16% 5=20% 6=24% 7=28% 8=32%
9=36% 10=40% 11=44% 12=48% 13=52% 14=56% 15=60%
16=64% 17=68% 18=72% 19=76% 20=80% 21=84% 22=88%
23=92% 24=96% 25=100%

Table 06.04

Questions for the 7-Day Quick Fix

1. You are desperate to lose a maximum of 7 pounds of fat very quickly
2. You are willing to follow a very strict food plan for one week
3. You understand that the maximum time on this plan is one week
4. You are willing to eat at home or at very specific places for one week
5. You are not taking any form of diabetic medication
6. You will complete at least 45 minutes per day of cardiovascular exercise for the week
7. You are 100% committed and will allow nothing short of an act of God to "derail" you
8. You have no gastrointestinal complaints (gas, bloating, heartburn, diarrhea, etc.)
9. You are between the ages of 15 and 60 years
10. You will begin another plan from this book right after this diet (no yo-yo dieting allowed)

Required # of yes answers = 10

Table 06.05

Questions for the Unlimited Protein
and Vegetables Plan

1. You often eat too much, unable to stop when you are full
2. You are very water retentive
3. You feel that you are addicted to sugar and/or carbohydrates
4. You feel fatigued most of the time
5. You like the idea of being able to eat certain foods in unlimited amounts
6. You are not a vegetarian (increased amount of protein makes plan difficult for vegetarians)
7. You will often feel abdominal bloating after a meal
8. You have had yeast infections (women) or jock itch (men) or athletes foot (men & women)
9. You do not urinate more than three times per day
10. You fall asleep within a few moments of laying your head on the pillow
11. You have high cholesterol, triglycerides, or blood pressure
12. You feel you may have food sensitivities/allergies
13. You have daily bowel movements (or you are starting a program to correct any GI troubles)
14. Your hair is thinning
15. Your nails are weak, peeling
16. You have dry, flaky skin
17. You have had more than one cold or flu in the last twelve months
18. You have large fat deposits in specific, concentrated areas
19. You have dieted in the past with little or no success
20. It has been at least one month since you have been on a strict diet

# of yes answers = ___6___ out of 20

% of yes answers ___30%___

1=5% 2=10% 3=15% 4=20% 5=25% 6=30% 7=35% 8=40%
9=45% 10=50% 11=55% 12=60% 13=65% 14=70% 15=75%
16=80% 17=85% 18=90% 19=95% 20=100%

Table 06.06

Questions for the Insulin Buster Plan

1. Does diabetes run in your family?
2. Have you had a very difficult time sticking to any sort of diet?
3. Do you have a large amount of fat around your abdomen (men) or your hips and thighs (women)?
4. Do you have overpowering cravings for carbohydrates?
5. Do you urinate frequently, even though you do not drink all that much?
6. Are you excessively thirsty?
7. Do you sometimes become sleepy after meals?
8. Do you awaken more than one time per night because of a need to urinate?
9. Do you have at least 25 pounds of fat to lose?
10. Do you often desire something sweet right after eating?
11. Do you have anxiety?
12. Are you shaped like an orange?
13. Do you have an ability to eat more than normal amounts of food?
14. Is your energy level like a roller coaster ride?
15. Does exercise or activity make you hungry?
16. Lightheadedness?
17. Weakness?
18. Water retention?
19. Do you have swollen legs and or feet?
20. Athletes foot or toenail fungus?
21. Yeast infections and or jock itch?
22. Dark circles under eyes?
23. Do you eat many of your meals away from home?
24. Do you like fatty foods?
25. Do you often wake up in the middle of the night hungry?

# of yes answers = ____7____ out of 25

% of yes answers ____28%____

1=4% 2=8% 3=12% 4=16% 5=20% 6=24% 7=28% 8=32%
9=36% 10=40% 11=44% 12=48% 13=52% 14=56% 15=60%
16=64% 17=68% 18=72% 19=76% 20=80% 21=84% 22=88%
23=92% 24=96% 25=100%

Table 06.07

Questions for the 40/40/20 Plan

1. You have at least 10 pounds of fat to lose
2. You have had some success with other diet plans in the past, and it took a while to regain the weight
3. You get mid-afternoon lows in your energy level
4. You sometimes have difficulty seeing at night
5. You often wake up with carbohydrate cravings
6. You feel anxiety when you go too long without food
7. You are forgetful
8. You get headaches
9. You sometimes feel faint
10. You will need to eat away from home at least a few times per week
11. You are between 15 and 60 years of age
12. Clammy skin
13. You get depressed
14. You love to eat breads
15. You have gained weight that you don't understand in the past few months
16. You are sometimes fatigued when you awaken
17. Excessive urination
18. Mild exercise causes fatigue
19. You have high blood pressure
20. Exercise has caused minimal changes in your appearance

# of yes answers = __13__ out of 20

% of yes answers __65%__

1=5% 2=10% 3=15% 4=20% 5=25% 6=30% 7=35% 8=40%
9=45% 10=50% 11=55% 12=60% 13=65% 14=70% 15=75%
16=80% 17=85% 18=90% 19=95% 20=100%

Table 06.08

Questions for the 50/30/20 Plan

1. Do you have fairly consistent energy levels?
2. You are active, spending more than 4 hours per week exercising
3. You have had a fairly easy time losing fat in the past, but do not keep it off
4. You sleep soundly at night
5. Your thirst is easily satisfied
6. Your body-fat percentage is close to where you want it to be
7. You have not had to diet much in the past
8. You do not get serious sugar cravings
9. One of your family members has diabetes
10. You sometimes feel warm when others are cold
11. You are fairly muscular
12. The last time you were on a diet was at least one month ago
13. Your body-fat is distributed evenly
14. You become full easily and your fullness lasts at least a few hours
15. You have lost all your fat and are now ready to go on a maintenance plan

# of yes answers = _____ out of 15

% of yes answers ___46%___

1= 7% 2=13% 3=20% 4=27% 5=33% 6=40% 7=46% 8=53%
9=60% 10=66% 11=73% 12=79% 13=86% 14=93% 15=100%

Table 06.09

Questions for the 30/50/20 Plan

1. You feel that carbohydrate containing foods make you gain weight
2. You have severe cravings for sweets
3. You have at least 10 pounds of fat to lose
4. You awaken in the night often, restless and agitated
5. You have tried other diets in the past and had little or no results
6. You have not been on a diet for at least one month (wait to start if you have—eat normally for one month)
7. Your body-fat is concentrated in the midsection (men) or hips and thighs (women)
8. You have or someone in your family has diabetes
9. You feel bloated and swollen
10. Your joints are achy
11. You do not recover from exercise quickly
12. You have acne
13. Your energy is unpredictable, it goes up and down without apparent reason
14. Your brain often feels "foggy"
15. You are willing to exercise once per week or more
16. Your socks often leave indents on your legs
17. You are willing to restrict your diet considerably to lose the fat
18. You are not a vegetarian (if vegetarian, protein will make plan difficult for you)
19. You will be able to eat at least 65% of your meals at home
20. You often feel dissatisfied with meals
21. You have high cholesterol
22. You have high blood pressure
23. You feel hungry after fruit
24. You do best when eating smaller, more frequent meals
25. You have high triglycerides

# of yes answers = ___8___ out of 25

% of yes answers __32%__

1=4% 2=8% 3=12% 4=16% 5=20% 6=24% 7=28% 8=32%
9=36% 10=40% 11=44% 12=48% 13=52% 14=56% 15=60%
16=64% 17=68% 18=72% 19=76% 20=80% 21=84% 22=88%
23=92% 24=96% 25=100%

Table 06.10

Questions for the Hi/Lo Plan

1. You have a deadline by which you must lose at least 5 pounds of fat
2. You are willing to do whatever it takes to lose the fat within this time
3. You have not been on a very low calorie diet for at least two weeks
4. You have had difficulty losing weight in the recent past
5. Dieting has always made you crave sugar
6. You are willing and able to eat very specific foods and amounts
7. You are willing and able to do at least 60 minutes of exercise at least 4 times per week
8. You are "stuck"—the diet that you chose (from this book) worked well at first, but has stopped working
9. You have lost all the fat, except in a very specific area (this area is not responding)
10. Your level of commitment is 100% (you will give up whatever you must to meet your goal)

Required number of yes answers = 8
Or, yes to numbers 8, 9, & 10

# of yes answers _____

## 7

THE UNLIMITED PROTEIN & VEGETABLES PLAN

EASE

As you would guess from the title of this chapter, you will not be eating carbohydrates while you are on this plan. Once you understand what it is you need to do. Once you explore your surroundings to determine where and when you can get the food that you need . . . this program becomes much easier.

EATING OUT

Eating out on this program can be very easy or it can be excruciatingly difficult, depending on how you approach it. The food selections on this nutritional program are protein and vegetables. If you look at any menu with the thought that you can't have any carbohydrates, you will find this to be difficult. If instead, you look at the menu and see all the options that you *do* have that include protein and vegetables, you will have no problem at all. Couple this with the fact that there are no limitations on how much or how frequently you eat, and this becomes a very easy program to accommodate while eating out. You will have to be somewhat selective about where you eat and/or how you order your meal. You will often find that particular attention must be paid to the manner in which your food is prepared. Foods must be free of undesirable carbohydrates. On occasion, a patient has done this program to the letter, and not had the dramatic results anticipated. When we examined their food choices, the main culprit was hidden carbohydrates that came in the form of food additives. So I must stress that you should pay close attention to the menu when you are eating out. Again, once you are "in the flow" of this program, it will be very easy to eat out.

RATE OF FAT LOSS

The rate of fat loss while you are on this program is usually very fast. I have seen patients lose up to 5 pounds of body-fat in a week. Your success will be determined by how frequently you eat and by your level of adherence to the rules. If you are following this program 50% of the time, you will have little or no result. If you follow it 80% of the time or better, you will have phenomenal results. Typical results are 2–5 pounds of fat loss per week

ENERGY

Starting with Day 1, you will have the best energy you have probably ever felt. From your first meal forward, you will be triggering great changes to your metabolism. These changes will result in increased energy levels, and this high energy will remain consistent, as long as you continue eating enough.

DURATION

The length of time that you stay on this program will be determined by your results, **but** *should not exceed six months in any case*. At some point while you are on this plan, you will reach a plateau. In other words, you will be losing fat, you will be feeling great, and everything will seem to be going really well—then three or four weeks will go by with no result. This is your goal. It will be at that time you will have remedied the hormonal imbalance you are striving to correct. Then it will be time to re-visit the "Is This You?" portion of the book (previous chapter) to decide what to do next.

YOUR UNIQUE METABOLISM

In finding your way to this food plan, you have found what may be the only diet that has the potential to bring your metabolism back to health. Because of your past dietary inconsistencies and imbalances, you have ended up with significant hormonal dismay.

But now, by following the unlimited protein and vegetables plan, you can recover—you can bring order to a disordered metabolism.

By answering "yes" to the "Is This You?" questions for this plan, you have discovered what is happening to the hormones that make up your metabolism. Your body is sending signals, trying to tell you it needs help. Help is on the way.

Your profile suggests that you have activated your starvation-protection mechanism. In other words, your body believes it is starving to death. The hormones and enzymes in your body that protect you against starvation are going crazy. It is likely that much of any food you eat will be turned into fat and stored away. (See Chapter 1.) In order to lose an ounce of fat, you will first have to turn off this protection circuit. In addition, it seems likely that you have elevated levels of adrenaline and cortisol. Elevations of these hormones make it impossible to feel or look your best. Elevations in adrenaline and cortisol also cause a cascade of other hormonal shifts, and this results in even more problems within the body. Apparently, the imbalances in your diet have also caused your cells to react differently to the hormones insulin and glucagon. This points to trouble ahead if you do not remedy this potentially serious imbalance.

The unlimited protein and vegetables plan will effectively reverse much of this chaos. This plan has been in my arsenal for many years and I have used it with hundreds of my clients. The plan works in a number of ways:

1. Increased frequency of meals will shut off starvation-protection mechanism.
2. Absence of carbohydrates will lower insulin levels.
3. Frequent intake of proteins and vegetables will cause ideal level of glucagon.
4. Frequent intake of protein and high nutrient intake form multivitamin/mineral/antioxidant will lower cortisol.
5. Shutting off starvation mechanism will lower adrenaline and cortisol levels.
6. Minimal level of fat intake will stimulate more hunger, which will cause you to eat more proteins, which will fuel your metabolism, and aid the above-mentioned mechanisms.

These major principles, and the many other reactions that this plan offers, spell relief for your body.

The type of problems you are experiencing are common. Your metabolism, however, is uncommon. It will take a unique approach to help you over this hurdle. I have created this plan precisely for you.

You will have tremendous success on this program.
Are you ready to transform your body?

THE PLAN

This nutritional program is very simple. You can eat as much protein, and as many vegetables (with the exception of carrots, peas, beets, squash, and corn) as you want, in any quantity, as often as you want. The object is to fuel the metabolism, and to give the metabolism only these foods so you can overcome your hormonal imbalances.

There are only two rules on this plan:

1. **You must eat enough protein and vegetables**. If you break this rule, you will fail. The word "enough" refers to the amount that is required to prevent hunger and cravings. If you are hungry, you must eat. If you get hungry and fail to eat within about twenty minutes, you will shut off all fat loss. One of the key points of this plan is to override your starvation-protection mechanism. The only way you will accomplish this is to eat large amounts of protein and veggies on a consistent basis. If you eat a piece of fish at 3:00 and you are hungry again at 4:00, you must eat again. It is easy to undereat, and **nearly impossible to overeat while on this plan**.

2. **On this plan you will completely avoid carbohydrates**. Carbohydrates are wreaking havoc on your body, and they *must* be avoided. They are the enemy. The only carbohydrates you consume will come from the list of "free foods." These are on the list specifically because they will have no significant effects on your blood-sugar level, and will not stimulate any significant production of insulin or imbalance any of the hormones that make up your metabolism. You may eat any food from the "free foods" list that you desire at any time. The endless variety of food, the frequency of feedings, and the fact that these foods do not have to be weighed or measured, make this a very easy plan, once you get in the groove.

When you are in the groove, you will find that you are hungry a lot, if not all the time. The idea is to eat as much protein as frequently as you can—all day—every day. You must eat when you are hungry. If you are not eating 5 or 6 times a day, you are not eating enough protein. You need that protein in your bloodstream at all times to maintain that hormonal balance that must occur in order for you to lose any body-fat. You will find that you are always eating something. Once you get into this groove, it is a self-propelling cycle. Your hunger will be stimulated by the intake of protein, and your hunger will demand that you eat more protein to satisfy that hunger.

When eating only protein while keeping the fat and carbohy-drate intake as low as they will be on this plan, it is very easy for your total caloric intake to go too low. If it does go too low, you will have activated your starvation-protection mechanism, which only causes the further secretion of insulin and imbalances between the other hormones. So it is very important that you eat frequently. If you have a chicken breast, and you are feeling hungry 15 minutes later, you must eat 15 minutes later. You *must* satisfy your hunger each and every time you are hungry. This will insure that you do not activate your starvation-protection mechanism.

Table 07.01

Acceptable Foods for the Unlimited Protein and Vegetables Plan

Proteins	**Vegetables**

<table>
<tr><td>

Proteins

Cook all proteins without fat.
Turkey breast
Chicken breast
Beefalo
Buffalo
Fish
Shellfish
Venison
Veal
Lamb
Ham
Canadian bacon
Lean steaks
7% fat ground beef
Lean cuts of pork
Egg whites
Egg substitute
Nonfat cottage cheese
Nonfat cheese
Tofu/Soy protein products
  (no carbs)
Protein powders: microfiltered,
  ion-exchanged, predigested
  whey is best.

</td><td>

Vegetables

Any vegetables, any amount.
  (Except corn, peas, squash,
   beets, and carrots)

</td></tr>
</table>

Table 07.02

Free Foods List

The following foods are free foods. Unless otherwise noted, you can consume them at any time, with or without meals.

All vegetables *Except corn, peas, squash, carrots, beets*
Diet sodas *Avoid those containing phosphoric acid or caffeine or saccharin*
Diet flavored waters *Avoid those containing phosphoric acid or caffeine or saccharin*
Crystal Light
Regular coffee *Up to 2 cups per day*
Unlimited decaffeinated coffee *Preferably water processed*
Herbal teas *Caffeine-free*
Iced tea *Sugar-free; avoid saccharin; decaffeinated; green tea is best*
Swiss Miss diet cocoa *Up to 2 packets per day*
Sugar-free Jell-o
Sugar-free gum
Frozen yogurt *Maximum 4 oz., 2 times per week*
Gise Frozen Yogurt (800) 448-4473
Nonfat sour cream
Nonfat cream cheese
Nonfat mayonnaise
Nonfat salad dressing *Maximum of 2 tbsp. per day*
Citrus peels
Vinegars
Lemon and lime juice
Extracts
All dry seasonings and herbal seasonings
BBQ, Teriyaki, Mustard, Relish, Salsa, Ketchup, A-1,
Soy sauce (low sodium)

Note: Consumption of aspartame-containing food products is a personal decision. Much data exists to support its safety, but this continues to be a much-debated issue.

YOUR FIRST WEEK

It is an understatement to say that during your first week your body will be going through significant changes. You will be restoring balance to what may have been unbalanced for most of your life. You may have never in your life arrived at what is correct for you, and that may be why you are reading this book. During this first week, you will be "kickstarting" your metabolism. As a result, you may be feeling certain things that are unusual for you. You may be depressed, or you may feel euphoric. You may get some acne, or you may eliminate the acne that you have. Your energy may soar, keeping you up at night, or you may feel totally lethargic for the first week. You will go through a number of metabolic changes that will result in symptoms that cannot be predicted. The only symptoms that should concern you are those that involve pain, disorientation, or discomfort. Consult your physician immediately if you have any concern.

You must keep moving forward, no matter what. No matter how you feel. I liken this to the way you would drive a car. You place your foot on the gas pedal, and the car begins to move forward. If you hold the gas pedal down, the car travels faster and faster. As the car travels faster, it also uses up more fuel. This fuel consumption allows the car to travel even faster. What happens when you let your foot off the gas pedal? The car slows back down. In other words, if you deprive yourself of food, you will not have enough gas fueling your engine. If, because you feel that you are eating too much, or eating foods that don't make sense, you change your plan in any way, *you will never get over the hump*. You will never reach freeway speeds, and you will be stuck on side-streets forever. So keep going forward, no matter what. For this first week, you will have to go on faith. Don't let up, and you will be well along on your journey.

HELPFUL HINTS

You must eat enough. This point cannot be made too force-fully. If you have been feeling hunger for more than the last twenty minutes, it's too late. Your metabolism has already gone into star-vation mode, and you're not losing any fat. Eat as much as it takes, as often as it takes.

You've heard it a hundred times, but I'll say it again. You must drink enough water. If you are dehydrated, you will not burn fat. End of story. Water is necessary in the process, not only of fat reduction, but every metabolic process as well. If you are not drinking enough water, you will fail. You should be urinating about ten times per day for your fat to remove itself from your body. If you are not in the bathroom more than you think you should be, you are not there often enough. Drink at least eight 12-oz. glasses of water each day.

For this or any other plan, preparation is key. Know that if you will be in the middle of nowhere when mealtime rolls around, you will have brought something to eat with you. If you know that you will be in the middle of a meeting when mealtime comes around, bring a meal replacement with you, so that you do not activate your starvation—protection mechanism. You don't have to eat a meal; you just have to ingest the proper amounts of carbohy-drate, protein, and fat. Prepare a thermos full of a meal replace-ment drink, to have throughout the day. Don't go out into the world everyday, and just expect that the right food will be there. It won't be. Think ahead. Plan for your success.

Take finger foods with you. Take easy-to-eat foods such as nonfat cheese sticks, protein shakes, turkey jerky, nonfat cottage cheese, etc. The more prepared you are, the greater your success will be.

Keep your fat intake low, but there is no need to go fat-free. If you order an item that has been bathed in a fattening sauce, just scrape it off. If you know your fish was cooked in butter, just scrape off the extra. When cooking at home, use the absolute minimal amount of oil. Use Teflon pans and cook things in their own juices.

You do not need to avoid fat like a disease, but on the other hand, don't get too friendly with fat, either.

It is most beneficial to have vegetables with each meal. Vegetables will not only eliminate any trace of carbohydrate craving, but will also be filling, and will regulate the bowels successfully. In addition to these benefits, many vegetables are high in the EFAs and contain special nutrients that are tremendously beneficial to the human body.

Do not have more than two alcoholic beverages per week. If you have a couple (two) glasses of alcohol per week, it should have no effect. Your body will absorb it, and you won't even see it. Any greater alcohol consumption becomes a ball and chain wrapped around your waist that you drag with you 24 hours a day. The alcoholic portion of any beverage you consume *will* be converted to body-fat. For women, this body-fat is gathered at the back of the arms, the hips, and just below the belly button. For men, it seems to gather between the chest and the pelvic area.

The correct supplementation program can dramatically enhance your results. My experience with thousands of clients has proven that the proper diet combined with a well-designed supplementation program will provide an average of approximately 30% *increased rate of fat reduction.* In addition to faster and greater fat reduction, you can achieve a stronger immune system, higher energy levels, and most important, a higher success rate of maintenance. You will find a comprehensive guide to these supplements in Chapter 5.

Get it? It's really that easy.

## 8

THE SUPER EFA PLAN

EASE

*T*he Super EFA is an aggressive approach to bringing balance back to the hormones that make up your metabolism. This plan will be a bit tricky for the first few days. When you overcome the main challenge of providing yourself with the proper food choices for this nutritional program, you will discover that it is truly easy to adhere to, and the benefits you will reap from this plan will be dramatic.

EATING OUT

Eating out will be either very easy or excruciatingly difficult, depending on your mindset. On this particular program, there are no allowances for carbohydrates. When you look at any restaurant menu with thoughts of sacrifice, this may be a difficult plan. However, if you can see the limitless choices that you *do* have, you will understand that you are really not sacrificing anything. When you can make this mental adjustment, you will find this plan to be extremely easy to adhere to while eating out.

RATE OF FAT REDUCTION

This plan might not be easy at first, and O.K., you can't have any carbohydrates . . . but the tradeoff in this case is a very significant reduction of body-fat. I have seen patients lose 7 pounds of body-fat in a week, and many others lose more than 15 pounds of body-fat in 20 days. You should expect to lose 2–6 pounds of body-fat per week.

ENERGY

While you are on this plan, you will feel a significant increase in energy. This surge will enable you to see dramatic improvements in your productivity and stamina. You will feel a sense of mental clarity that may have been nonexistent or missing for a very long time, and in turn, this will make you even more productive and insightful. You may also notice a major improvement in skin tone, hair quality, stronger nails, and a heightened level of wellness that you have not been feeling in a long while.

DURATION

This is a temporary plan, designed to remedy a problem that demands fixing. The Super EFA is a plan that focuses on correcting a specific set of deficiencies. Usually the process of correcting your essential fatty acid deficiency would take no more than 60 days. At the end of this 60-day period, your metabolism will be vastly different, and you will have a completely different set of needs. You should then return to the "Is This You?" questions in Chapter 6, to determine what to do next.

YOUR UNIQUE METABOLISM

By answering "yes" to the majority of questions within the "Is This You?" section regarding the Super EFA Plan, you have indicated that you have had a significant deficiency of essential fatty acids within your body for quite a while. In addition to balancing the hormones that make up your body's metabolism, and in addition to gaining control over your caloric intake, you will also have to reverse your deficiency in essential fatty acids to achieve more energy, wellness, and lasting fat reduction.

Essential fatty acids are special fats that your body requires. They are called essential fatty acids because it is *essential* that you derive them from your diet. Unlike other substances, these fatty acids cannot be manufactured your body. These essential fatty acids are found in many different foods. These foods are the basis for this plan.

Because you have a deficiency of these essential fatty acids, many areas of the body and functions of the metabolism become dysfunctional. Your wellness may indeed suffer, and over time, you will become prone to a number of diseases including, cancer, diabetes, cardiovascular diseases, and obesity. There can also be a number of lesser discomforts also associated with a deficiency in essential fatty acids, such as psoriasis, eczema, early menopause for women, early andropause for men, infertility for both sexes, neurological disorders, arthritis, and numerous other problems.

By following the diet that is detailed in this chapter, you will be able to reverse this deficiency within your body and overcome the likelihood of acquiring these illnesses and diseases, and certainly have the ability to shed a significant amount of body-fat.

This deficiency in essential fatty acids has had a ripple effect throughout the hormones that govern your metabolism, and there may even be indications that you are beginning to develop insensitivity to the hormone, insulin. This phenomenon can set off a chain of events that are detrimental to the reduction of body-fat, and your overall health in general. As an indirect result of this insulin resistance, glucagon levels are lower than they should be. This causes an over-secretion of cortisol, which in turn limits production of human growth hormone. This hormonal imbalance takes over. Although this basic hormonal imbalance is relatively common, your body is unique and so requires a unique approach to bring it to health.

Your unique metabolism will need an extra injection or boost to strike the ideal balance. By increasing the amount of *good* fat you will eat, the essential fatty acids that are now severely deficient will be brought back to normal levels. At the same time as you increase the amount of protein you eat, you will also eliminate carbohydrates.

This combination will allow insulin and glucagon to be equally balanced, which in turn, will allow all the other hormones to line up properly. By eating in this way, you will also positively affect your *future health*. This way of eating may reduce your risk of cancer, heart disease, stroke, diabetes and, of course, obesity. Your energy will go up immediately, and remain absolutely stable. You will no longer experience the ups and downs in your energy during the day, and may in fact, feel more vital than you have ever felt. This will all take place as a result of the increased intake of essential fatty acids and by bringing a balance to the hormones.

The process of correcting your essential fatty acid deficiency will take no more than 60 days. Either at the end of the 60 days, or if at any time during the 60 days, you feel that you have reached a plateau, return to the "Is This You?" questions to determine what to do next.

THE PLAN

This aggressive plan is a high-protein, high-fat, and very low-carbohydrate approach to fat reduction and wellness. Fat is seen by most as the enemy. In my professional opinion, the bad "rap" that fat has received by the medical community is unwarranted. In your case, fat is definitely not the enemy. On this nutritional program, the high-fat intake you will have is absolutely healthy fat. These fats are essential to the human body and, in no case, or in any conceivable way, could they or will they be "bad" for you. For you, there cannot be significant body-fat reduction without first correcting your deficiency of essential fatty acids. Once this deficiency has been reversed, balance will return to the hormones that make up the metabolism, and other systems in the body and you will achieve a level of fat reduction and vitality.

I know what you're asking yourself. You are saying, "Wait, how do I get thin from eating fat?" You have probably learned in the past that fat makes you fat. Nothing could be further from the truth. Fat does not, nor does it have the potential to, make you fat. Insulin makes you fat. Hormonal imbalances make you fat. Fat does not promote the production of insulin. Carbohydrates have much more potential to create body-fat than fat does. Surprisingly, this particular diet also has benefited a large majority of individuals who suffer from high blood pressure, diabetes, and high cholesterol levels. The food combination of this diet focuses on protein and good fats. When you consume good fat and protein together there is very little insulin production. Therefore, dietary fat cannot be converted into body-fat but instead, it is used to fuel the body.

The first step in getting started on your new plan is to determine the approximate number of calories you will need to eat each meal, each day.

On the following pages you will find the formulas needed to make these calculations.

Take a few moments and fill in the blanks. I recommend that you actually write in the book and use it like a workbook.

Once you have made the necessary calculations, we will go on and apply them to the food list and determine what your meals will look like.

YOUR BODY'S ENERGY (CALORIE) REQUIREMENTS

Basal Energy Requirement (BER)

The first step in designing your personal nutritional program is to determine your basal energy requirement (BER). The BER is the amount of energy your body requires in order to fuel its most basic functions. The BER is the approximate number of calories needed to breathe, think, pump blood through veins, etc.

There will be two different formulas for the BER. One for those who have had their body-fat measured, and one for those who have not. I strongly urge you to have your body-fat measured prior to starting your nutritional plan. The BER is much more accurately determined if you know your fat percentage. If you have not had your fat measured, skip this section and proceed to the next.

The first step in determining the BER is to determine the amount of lean body weight you have. As we discussed in Chapter 1, lean body weight is the amount of your body that is not fat. It is the portion of your body that is composed of muscle, organs, bones, water, and other nonfat tissues.

For those who know their body-fat percentage, the formula to determine the amount of lean body weight is as follows. If you have not had your body-fat measured, skip this and go to the next section.

Body weight _____ × Body-fat% _____ = Fat weight _____

Body weight _____ – Fat weight _____ = **Lean body weight (LBW)** _____

Example

A person who weighs 100 lbs. with a body-fat of 15% will have 15 pounds of fat. This person would then have 85 lbs. of lean body weight (100 – 15 = 85). Once you have determined your lean body weight (LBW), the next step is to factor in your age.

Age Factor

Now take your lean body weight (LBW) and *multiply it by your age factor.* You will then have your basal energy requirement (BER).

- 50 years or older, the age factor is 13
- 40–50 years, the age factor is 14
- 20–40 years, the age factor is 15
- Up to 20 years, the age factor is 16

For example, a person with a LBW of 100 lbs., who is 36 years old, will have a BER of 1500. (100 × 15 = 1500)

Now, calculate your own BER.

LBW _____ × age factor _____ = BER _____

Total Energy Requirement (TER)

Remember—the BER is the approximate number of calories your body will require to do nothing but exist. If you are active, you will need to adjust the BER to account for the energy expended during the activities. This number will be your total energy requirement or your TER. The total energy requirement is the approximate number of calories that your body will require to keep itself alive, and to perform the various activities of the day. In order to determine your TER, you will need to factor in your level of activity.

Activity Factor

The activity factor is used to approximate the number of calories you will need to consume to replace the amount of energy expended during exercise and other activities. Take your BER and add the appropriate number from the list below. If you are not active, skip this calculation.

- If you participate in up to 30 minutes of exercise/activity per day, multiply your LBW by 2.
- If you participate in 30–60 minutes of exercise/activity per day, multiply your LBW by 3.
- If you participate in 60–90 minutes of exercise/activity per day, multiply your LBW by 4.

Example

A person who has a BER of 1500 calories and a lean body weight of 100 lbs., who exercises 60 minutes per day (activity factor = LBW multiplied by 3) will end up with a number of 1800. BER 1500 + Activity factor 300 = 1800. This number is the TER, or total energy requirement.

Now calculate your own activity factor.

LBW = _____ × (2, 3, or 4) _____ = activity factor _____

Now determine your total energy requirement (TER).

BER = _____ + Activity factor _____ = TER _____

(If you are inactive, your BER is the same as your TER.)

Adjusted Total Energy Requirement (ATER)

Remember—the TER is the approximate number of calories you would consume in a day if you wanted to maintain your current status. However, if you want to lose some body-fat, you will need to give your body a reason to use the fat as fuel. With few exceptions, this is accomplished by reducing the caloric intake to well below what your body requires to do the day's work. This adjusted calorie amount is known as the adjusted total energy requirement (ATER). As long as all the hormones are doing their jobs, and your metabolism is in a state of balance, the significant deficit of energy will cause your body to go into its fat reserves to get the missing energy. Hence, a reduction in body-fat.

To calculate your adjusted total energy requirement (ATER), simply take your TER and subtract 500.

Example

TER 1800 – 500 = 1300. (1300 is the ATER)

Now calculate your own adjusted total energy requirement (ATER).

TER _____ – 500 = _____ ATER

This number reflects the approximate number of calories you need to consume each day while attempting to lose body-fat. When you have lost all the fat you want to lose, use your TER as your daily caloric intake.

ENERGY (CALORIE) REQUIREMENTS WITHOUT A BODY-FAT MEASUREMENT

Caution: These formulas are only 70% accurate without a measurement of your body-fat percentage. *I recommend that you have your body-fat measured as soon as possible.*

Estimated Total Energy Requirement (ETER)

The *estimated* total energy requirement (ETER) is the approximate amount of energy (calories) that your body will need in a day to perform its basic functions (such as breathing and thinking), *in addition to* what it will require to complete the usual amount of exercise/activity.

Use the following guide to determine your ETER.

STEP ONE IS TO MULTIPLY YOUR BODY WEIGHT BY YOUR WEIGHT FACTOR.

Weight Factor

The weight factor is an approximation of the total amount of energy (calories) that a person of your weight, with an average amount of body-fat would need in a day just to maintain normal body function, such as breathing, thinking, etc. Use the following list to determine your weight factor.

- **Women** who weigh up to 120 lbs—multiply your weight by *8.5*
- **Women** who weigh between 121 and 150 lbs.—multiply your weight by *8.25*
- **Women** who weigh between 151 and 200 lbs.—multiply your weight by *8*
- **Women** who weigh between 200 and 250 lbs.—multiply your weight by *7*
- **Women** who weigh more than 250 lbs.—multiply your weight by *6.5*
- **Men** who weigh up to 165 lbs.—multiply your weight by *10*
- **Men** who weigh 166 and 190 lbs.—multiply your weight by *9.5*
- **Men** who weigh more than 190 lbs.—multiply your weight by *9.25*

Now calculate your own weight factor.

Body weight _____ × _____ (weight factor) = _____

STEP TWO IS TO APPLY YOUR ACTIVITY FACTOR.

Activity Factor

The activity factor is used to approximate the number of calories you will need to consume to replace the amount of energy expended during exercise and other activities. Take your weight factor and add the appropriate number from the list below. If you are sedentary, skip this calculation.

- If you participate in up to 30 minutes of exercise/activity per day, add .5 calories per pound of body weight to your weight factor
- If you participate in 30–60 minutes of exercise/activity per day, add 1 calorie per pound of body weight to your weight factor
- If you participate in more than 60 minutes of exercise/activity per day, add 1.5 calories per pound of body weight to your weight factor

Example

A male who weighs 176 lbs. has a weight factor of 1672 (176 × 9.5 = 1672).

If he exercises 60 minutes per day, he has an activity factor of 176 (1 cal × 176 lbs. = 176).

So, his estimated total energy requirement (ETER) would be 1848 (1672 + 176 = 1848).

Now, calculate your own ETER.

Weight factor _____ + Activity factor _____ = _____ *ETER*

YOUR IDEAL EFA MEAL

Let's now determine how you should split that total caloric intake up to arrive at your ideal EFA meal, which for you is: **55% protein and 45% Fat**.

You begin with your adjusted total energy requirement (ATER), or your *estimated* total energy requirement (ETER), and divide that by 4. This number will represent the approximate number of calories that are reserved for each meal.

ATER or ETER _____ ÷ 4 = _____ calories per meal

You will have *4* meals of _____ calories each.

If you have 1000 calories per day, you would divide that number of calories by 4 to determine the calories for each meal. (1000 divided by four = 250 calories in each of these segments.) Three of these segments would be reserved for breakfast, lunch, a mid-afternoon meal, dinner, and the last meal—two hours before bedtime. Each of these meals would be 250 calories each.

Lets now split up each meal into the portion of 55% & 45%.

Calories per meal _____ × 55%(.55) = _____ protein *calories* per meal

Because protein contains 4 calories per gram, you will need to divide that number buy 4 to determine the ideal number of grams of protein per meal.

Protein calories per meal _____ ÷ 4 = _____ **grams of protein per meal**

Calories per meal _____ × 45%(.45) = _____ fat *calories* per meal

Because fat contains 9 calories per gram, you will need to divide that number by 9 to determine the ideal number of grams of fat per meal.

Fat calories per meal _____ ÷ 9 = _____ **grams of fat per meal**

I'm sure you're asking yourself, "Yeah, so what does that mean to me?" You have now successfully determined the proper amounts of proteins and fats for each meal. Now it is time to put that knowledge into practice. On the following page you will find a food list. This is the list of acceptable foods for the Super EFA.

The Super EFA requires that you eat **4 equally balanced meals per day.** It is the most critical component of the plan. You must not eat less than 4 meals per day, no matter what. Each of these meals should be spaced about four hours apart (3–5 is the window). Each meal, you simply choose a protein and a fat selection, and calculate the appropriate amounts of those foods, using the formulas, and checking the food list to figure out the amount that you need to have. For instance, lets say that you have determined that you need 35 grams of protein for each meal, and you will be eating chicken breasts tonight. Looking at the food list, you will see that chicken has 7 grams of protein per ounce. This would mean that you would need 5 ounces of chicken to satisfy the protein requirements for your ideal Super EFA meal. You may split the portions. In other words, you can have half the correct amount of chicken, and half the correct amount of egg whites together, to add up to one full portion. You can also do this with the fat portion of your meal.

The "free foods" are allowed at any time, with or without meals, as ingredients in recipes, fillers, snacks, or however you want to use them.

On the following page you will find a food list. This list contains all of the foods that are allowed on the Super EFA. If you do not see it on the list, the answer is no.

Table 08.01

Super EFA Food List

PROTEIN	FAT	FREE FOODS	BEVERAGES
*Chicken breast	Sunflower oil	All vegetables *except*	Diet sodas
*Turkey breast	Hemp oil	**Corn, peas, carrots**	*Avoid phosphoric acid*
*Fish	Soybean oil	**Squash, beets**	Crystal light
*Shellfish	Olive oil	Sugar free Jell-o	Diet flavored waters
7% fat ground beef	Safflower oil	Sugar free gum	2 cups reg. Coffee
Lean steak	Canola oil	Gise Frozen Yogurt	Unlimited decaf coffee
	4 grams fat per tsp.		Herbal teas
Veal			Iced tea
Lamb			*(sugar free, preferably decaf)*
Pork	Avocado		
Venison	*3 grams fat/oz.*		
Buffalo			
Beefalo	Olives		**CONDIMENTS:**
average 7 grams protein/oz.	*Average 1 gram fat ea.*		Nonfat sour cream
			Nonfat Cream cheese
*Egg whites	Nut Butters		Nonfat Mayonnaise
3 grams protein ea.	*(I.E. Peanut butter, Almond butter, etc)*		Nonfat salad dressing
	3 grams protein per tsp.		BBQ/Teriyaki sauce
Nonfat cottage cheese	Nuts		Salsa
Average 3 grams protein/oz.	*Check fat content per oz.*		Relish
			Ketchup
	Seeds		Mustard
*Egg substitute	*Check fat content per oz.*		Steak sauce
Check label for protein content			Steak sauce
			Low salt soy sauce
Tofu			All dry seasonings
Check label for protein content			*Use Condiments sparingly*

*Protein powders
Check label for protein content
*Indicates best choices
All amounts listed are cooked.
Cook all proteins without fat.

YOUR FIRST WEEK

It is an understatement to say that during your first week, your body will be going through significant changes. You will be bringing back balance to what may have been unbalanced for most of your life. You may have never in your life arrived at what is correct for you. Because you are reading this book, you probably haven't. During this first week, you will be rearranging the metabolism. As a result, you may be feeling certain things that are unusual for you. You may be depressed, or you may feel euphoric. You may get some acne, or you may eliminate the acne that you have. Your energy may soar, keeping you up at night, or you may feel totally lethargic for the first week. You will go through a number of metabolic changes that will result in symptoms that I am not able to predict.

What you must do is keep moving forward, no matter what. No matter how you feel. I liken this to the way you would drive a car. You place your foot on the gas pedal, and the car begins to move forward. If you hold the gas pedal down, the car travels faster and faster. As the car travels faster, it also uses up more fuel. This fuel consumption allows the car to travel even faster. What happens when you let your foot off the gas pedal? The car slows back down. In other words, if you deprive yourself of food, you will not have enough gas in your engine. If you feel like you are eating too much, or eating foods that don't make sense, and you change your plan in any way, *you will never get over the hump*. You will never reach free-way speeds, and you will be stuck on side-streets forever. So keep going forward no matter what. For this first week you will have to go on faith. Don't let up, and you will be well on your journey.

HELPFUL HINTS

You must not miss meals. If you do not eat **four** times a day at least 80% of the time, you will not succeed.

If you happen to over-eat one meal, do not *under-eat during the next meal.* In other words, do not alter any meal, based on a mistake you made on the meal prior to that, or in anticipation of a meal that is ahead of you. By doing this you will have ruined *two* meals. Each meal is its own separate entity, that is not reliant on the other meal. Each meal is like taking a medicine that we are trying to get an effect from, that will wear off in a few hours, so we would take that medicine again. If you change the medicine once, would you change the medicine again to account for that? No. You can't double up, you can't cut it in half. You will simply be ruining a half of your day instead of a quarter of a day. Even in cases of extreme over-eating, the next meal is exactly as it should be. We are attempting to create an environment for your metabolism. Allow that environment to be as stable as possible.

You've heard it a hundred times, but I'll say it again. You **must** *drink enough water.* If you are dehydrated, you will not burn fat. End of story. Water is necessary in the process, not only of fat reduction, but every metabolic process as well. If you are not drinking enough water, you will fail. You should be urinating about ten times per day for your fat to remove itself from your body. If you are not in the bathroom more than you think you should be, you are not there often enough. Drink at least eight 12 oz. glasses of water each day.

Another suggestion I would make would be to purchase a food scale. Don't assume that you know anything, even if you have been on a program where you had to weigh your food. It is vital that you are getting the proper amount of food in the correct ratios for this to work for you. You don't want to be, and you don't need to be measuring everything that you eat. However, for the first week or so, I want you to get a better idea of what your portion size will look like. If you have determined, by using "The Perfect Portion," that you need 6 oz. of protein with each meal, weigh that out before and after cooking. Put it in your bowl of salad or on the plate, so that you can be accustomed to what that portion size looks like. Give yourself that edge, you'll thank me for it down the road.

For this or any other plan, preparation is key. Know that if you will be in the middle of nowhere when mealtime rolls around, that you will have brought something to eat with you. If you know that you will be in the middle of a meeting when mealtime comes around, bring a meal replacement with you, so that you do not activate your starvation-protection mechanism. You don't have to eat a meal; you just have to ingest the proper amounts of carbohydrate, protein, and fat. Prepare a thermos full of a meal replacement drink, to have throughout the day. Don't go out into the world everyday, and just expect that the right food will be there. It won't be. Think ahead. Plan for your success.

Make sure you are getting enough protein. Most menu items will not have the 55% protein content that you require. You must learn to order additional portions, or let them know exactly how much you need.

Foods that are highlighted by an * on the "food list" are optimal choices. If you choose to eat these highlighted foods 80% of the time, your results will improve by 40%.

Foods must be eaten together, at the same time, to attain the desired results. You must eat in this manner to repress or stimulate the various hormones that are out of balance within the metabolism. To activate the specific hormones, foods must be ingested together as a whole meal. Do not, under any circumstances, have a protein without the fat portion of the meal, and vice versa. These food groups must always be consumed at the same time, or eating in this prescribed manner will have the opposite outcome than the results you desire.

It is most beneficial to have vegetables with each meal. Vegetables will not only eliminate any trace of carbohydrate craving, but will also be filling, and will regulate the bowels successfully. In addition to these benefits, many vegetables are high in the EFAs and contain special nutrients that are tremendously beneficial to the human body.

Do not have more than two alcoholic beverages per week. If you have a couple (two) glasses of alcohol per week, it should have no effect. Any greater alcohol consumption becomes a ball and chain wrapped around your waist that you drag with you 24 hours a day. The alcoholic portion of any beverage you consume *will* be converted to body-fat. For women, this body-fat is gathered at the back of the arms, the hips and just below the belly button. For men, it seems to gather between the chest and the pelvic area.

The correct supplementation program can dramatically enhance your results. My experience with thousands of clients has proven that the proper diet combined with a well-designed supplementation program will provide an average of approximately *30% increased rate of fat reduction*. In addition to faster and greater fat reduction, you can achieve a stronger immune system, higher energy levels, and most important, a higher success rate of maintenance. You will find a comprehensive guide to these supplements in Chapter 5.

Meal replacement "Protein bars" are an excellent way to have a meal in a hurry or on-the-go. Depending on which plan you have chosen, you will be required to eat 4–7 times per day. In many cases, this is a difficult task, one that can be made much easier with the option of having a meal replacement bar. Just open the wrapper and eat your meal—it is as easy as that. You can use these bars as often as needed, as long as they contain the appropriate amounts of proteins, carbohydrates and fats. There are many of these bars available. The trick is to find the bar that contains the necessary amounts of proteins, carbohydrates, and fats for your plan. To find the right bar, just go to your local health food store and either look at the labels yourself, or ask for help. You can also call (888) 663-2881 to have some of the right bars sent to you.

You've got the tools, now put 'em to work!

## 9

THE PROTEIN PLUS ONE PLAN

EASE

*T*his is an extremely easy program to follow. This plan is moderate and accommodating, allowing unlimited meals and snacks consisting of protein and vegetable selections, along with one fairly large, unstructured "non-diet" meal per day.

EATING OUT

Since most of us choose to eat out for only one meal on any given day, this plan is an idyllic choice for those of us who do eat out. You are allowed one meal per day to eat whatever you want . . . with minimal restrictions.

RATE OF FAT LOSS

On this particular plan it is imperative to eat when you are hungry. The more frequently you eat, the faster your body-fat loss will be on this particular program. I have had clients lose over 30 pounds of body-fat in eight weeks on this program. The average loss is 2–3 pounds of body-fat per week.

ENERGY LEVEL

While following this plan your energy levels will remain high and consistent. You should have none of the usual mid-afternoon slumps, peaks and valleys, etc. You will wake up clear and feel tired only just before bedtime.

DURATION

By answering "yes" to the majority of "Is This You?" questions, you have indicated that this plan will work exceptionally well for your body. You may choose to adhere to the plan for the rest of your life. One could and should stay on this program for as long is it is effective.

THE PROTEIN PLUS ONE PLAN

The Protein Plus One plan is a high protein, low carbohydrate plan that I have designed for people *just like you*.

The Protein Plus One program will allow you to change the characteristics of your metabolism that are stopping you from achieving wellness and lasting fat reduction. Utilizing the Protein Plus One plan will enable you to shed the unwanted body-fat and pounds. This nutritional program will also *increase* your energy level while *decreasing* your risk of many diseases. These results will be permanent because you will correct the very hormonal imbalances that are at the heart of your problems. These hormones are intimately involved in the process of fat loss and must be balanced for any long-term success to take place. It is important to know that you are not doing something temporary here. While you are worried about the here and now, and would like to look and feel better today, it is of much greater concern what will happen tomorrow and next year. The Protein Plus One plan will not only get you through today and tomorrow but will insure that you stay thin and healthy for the long term.

YOUR UNIQUE METABOLISM

There are several unique characteristics of your metabolism that must be properly addressed in order for you to attain the goals that you have set. It is precisely these unique signature characteristics that have resulted in an increased level of body-fat, a decreased level of muscle, a less than optimal metabolism, and a propensity for obesity, diabetes, high blood pressure, and cardiovascular disease. We must correct these signature characteristics in order for you to feel, look, and be your best.

Your answers to the "Is This You?" portion of the book indicate that your body **does not** need a large amount of carbohydrates. When you consume too many carbohydrates relative to the level of your body's needs, it will cause certain hormonal imbalances that will lead to trouble. We must therefore keep the carbohydrate intake on your particular food plan at a relatively low level. Another trait of your metabolism is that you require a high level of protein intake. This can be difficult because we live in a very "high-carbohydrate society," which emphasizes foods like breads, pasta, and French fries. All of these carbohydrates are the easiest food to obtain, and they are everywhere within reach. In fact they are often the recommended food. Even the government's food pyramid, which is supposed to be universal to all people, recommends very high carbohydrate levels . . . and for you, **high carbohydrates guarantee your failure and lack of wellness.**

As a result of underconsuming protein and overconsuming carbohydrate, you will have an imbalance between certain hormones in your body. These hormones being insulin, human growth hormone, glucagon, and cortisol. These hormones have very important functions in your body and are very deeply involved in your energy, your wellness, your ability to reduce body-fat, disease prevention, etc. Needless to say, it would be in your best interest to balance these hormones in a favorable way. This will definitely *not* happen with a high-carbohydrate/low-protein intake.

Also your answers to the "Is This You?" portion of the book indicate that you have an **activated starvation protection mechanism**. This starvation mechanism is a protection circuit built into the human body that detects the amount of nutrient and calorie intake and compares it to the amount that is being expended. When the amount that is taken in is significantly less than the amount that is being put out, the body will slow down the rate at which it burns calories and nutrients. In other words, the body will conserve energy by storing the food you do eat into body-fat. Instead of using your food for fuel, your body will begin to burn less essential tissues to produce the energy needed to keep you going all day. These tissues include muscle, bone, and organs. Needless to say, this is not how you want to fuel your body. You must override this starvation-protection mechanism to get out of the metabolic rut that you are stuck in. The starvation-protection mechanism may be *deactivated* by eating consistent and frequent meals containing the proper food combinations.

All of these problems, these signature characteristics of your metabolism, can be overcome by significantly increasing your protein intake and decreasing your carbohydrate intake. This strategy for eating will not only increase the levels of growth hormone and glucagon, but will also lower the levels of insulin and cortisol, thereby reducing the risk for cardiovascular disease, obesity, high cholesterol, high triglycerides, and high blood pressure.

THE PLAN

The Protein Plus One plan is comprised of a *frequent* and *consistent* intake of protein throughout the day, plus one balanced carbohydrate-containing meal. This plan requires you to consume significant amounts of protein frequently and consistently throughout each and every day, with the knowledge that this protein will fuel your body. It will give your body the tools that it needs to overcome the hormonal imbalances and the starvation protection mechanism that we mentioned earlier.

THE OBJECT OF THE PROTEIN PLUS ONE PLAN IS TO CONSUME VAST AMOUNTS OF PROTEIN EACH DAY

The idea is to enhance your metabolism, which will only happen through the frequent and consistent consumption of protein. It is essential that you understand that the more protein you eat, the faster you will lose on this plan. You cannot overeat, and it is very easy to undereat on this plan. Begin each day with the intention of consuming as much protein as you possibly can, along with an unlimited amount of vegetables, and free foods. You must have only one meal per day containing carbohydrates.

Typically this carbohydrate-containing meal will be 50%–60% carbohydrates, 30%–40% protein, and 10%–20% fat. The actual amount of calories from this meal is not important. The size of the meal should be determined by the volume of food it takes for you to become satisfied. You should not feel stuffed or overfull after this meal. Favorable balance between carbohydrates and protein is absolutely critical. Fats on this plan should be kept to a minimum. This meal can be eaten at any time of the day or night, up until two hours before bedtime, and again, it is only *one* time per day that you will eat carbohydrates.

ONE IMPORTANT NOTE WHEN YOU ARE FOLLOWING THE PROTEIN PLUS ONE PLAN

When you are eating adequate amounts of protein, you will become satiated much more easily. When it comes time to eat the one meal containing carbohydrates, your appetite will be under control, you will receive the signals from your stomach that you are feeling full, and you will have the ability to stop eating at that time. Your current hormonal imbalances are not allowing these signals to be received properly and it is nearly impossible to discontinue eating when it is appropriate. If you are eating enough protein, everything will work perfectly. If you are not, you will crave carbohydrates, and find it nearly impossible to avoid them. You will have lagging energy, and you will not lose fat. One sure way to determine if you are consuming enough protein on a regular basis is whether or not you are craving carbohydrates. If you are, it signals that you are undereating protein.

Table 09.01

Protein Plus One Food List

PROTEINS   (*Unlimited amounts*)

Turkey breast*	Lean steaks	Venison*
Lean cuts of pork	Beefalo*	Canadian bacon
Buffalo	Nonfat cheese	Fish*
Nonfat cottage cheese	Shellfish*	Ham
Lamb	Egg substitute	Veal
Egg Whites*	7% fat ground beef	Protein powders* (Microfiltered, ion-exchanged, predigested whey protein is best.)
Chicken Breast		

CARBOHYDRATES   (*Once per day*)

Yams/Sweet Potatoes*	Breads	Red potatoes*
Bagels	Rice*	Corn tortillas
Oats*	Flour tortillas	Beans/Lentils*
Fruit	Melon	Pasta

Tofu/Soy protein products (Watch for extra carbs and fats.)

*Indicates best choices

Table 09.02

Free Foods List

The following foods are free foods. Unless otherwise noted, you can consume them at any time, with or without meals.

All vegetables *Except corn, peas, squash, carrots, beets*
Diet sodas *Avoid those containing phosphoric acid or caffeine or saccharin*
Diet flavored waters *Avoid those containing phosphoric acid or caffeine or saccharin*
Crystal Light
Regular coffee *Up to 2 cups per day*
Unlimited decaffeinated coffee *Preferably water processed*
Herbal teas *Caffeine-free*
Iced tea *Sugar-free; avoid saccharin; decaffeinated; green tea is best*
Swiss Miss diet cocoa *Up to 2 packets per day*
Sugar-free Jell-o
Sugar-free gum
Frozen yogurt *Maximum 4 oz., 2 times per week*
Gise Frozen Yogurt (800) 448-4473
Nonfat sour cream
Nonfat cream cheese
Nonfat mayonnaise
Nonfat salad dressing *Maximum of 2 tbsp. per day*
Citrus peels
Vinegars
Lemon and lime juice
Extracts
All dry seasonings and herbal seasonings
**BBQ, Teriyaki, Mustard, Relish, Salsa, Ketchup, A-1,
Soy sauce (low sodium)**

Note: Consumption of aspartame-containing food products is a personal decision. Much data exists to support its safety, but this continues to be a much-debated issue.

YOUR DAILY CARBOHYDRATE-CONTAINING MEAL

The graph below represents the average content of your daily carbohydrate-containing meal. The meal should be approximately 50% carbohydrate, 35% protein, and 15% fat. The number of calories is unimportant. Just maintain the balance, and do not overeat.

Graph 09.01

Your daily carbohydrate-containing meal

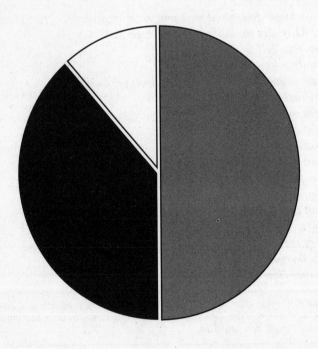

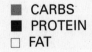

YOUR FIRST WEEK

It is an understatement to say that during your first week your body will be going through significant changes. You will be restoring balance to what may have been unbalanced for most of your life. You may have never in your life arrived at what is correct for you, and that may be why you are reading this book. During this first week, you will be "kickstarting" your metabolism. As a result, you may be feeling certain things that are unusual for you. You may be depressed, or you may feel euphoric. You may get some acne, or you may eliminate the acne that you have. Your energy may soar, keeping you up at night, or you may feel totally lethargic for the first week. You will go through a number of metabolic changes that will result in symptoms that cannot be predicted. The only symptoms that should concern you are those that involve pain, disorientation, or discomfort. Consult your physician immediately if you have any concern.

You must keep moving forward, no matter what. No matter how you feel. I liken this to the way you would drive a car. You place your foot on the gas pedal, and the car begins to move forward. If you hold the gas pedal down, the car travels faster and faster. As the car travels faster, it also uses up more fuel. This fuel consumption allows the car to travel even faster. What happens when you let your foot off the gas pedal? The car slows back down. In other words, if you deprive yourself of food, you will not have enough gas fueling your engine. If, because you feel that you are eating too much, or eating foods that don't make sense, you change your plan in any way, *you will never get over the hump*. You will never reach freeway speeds, and you will be stuck on side-streets forever. So keep going forward, no matter what. For this first week, you will have to go on faith. Don't let up, and you will be well along on your journey.

HELPFUL HINTS

You must not miss meals. If you do not eat four times a day, at least 80% of the time, you will not succeed.

You've heard it a hundred times, but I'll say it again. You must drink enough water. If you are dehydrated, you will not burn fat. End of story. Water is necessary in the process, not only of fat reduction, but every metabolic process as well. If you are not drinking enough water, you will fail. You should be urinating about ten times per day for your fat to remove itself from your body. If you are not in the bathroom more than you think you should be, you are not there often enough. Drink at least eight 12-oz. glasses of water each day.

For this or any other plan, preparation is key. Know that if you will be in the middle of nowhere when mealtime rolls around, that you will have brought something to eat with you. If you know that you will be in the middle of a meeting when mealtime comes around, bring a meal replacement with you, so that you do not activate your starvation-protection mechanism. You don't have to eat a meal; you just have to ingest the proper amounts of carbohydrate, protein, and fat. Prepare a thermos full of a meal replacement drink, to have throughout the day. Don't go out into the world everyday, and just expect that the right food will be there. It won't be. Think ahead. Plan for your success.

Make sure you are getting enough protein. Most menu items will not have the protein content that you require. You must learn to order additional portions, or let them know exactly how much you need. On this plan, failure to consume enough protein guarantees your failure

It is most beneficial to have vegetables with each meal. Vegetables will not only eliminate any trace of carbohydrate craving, but will also be filling, and will regulate the bowels successfully. In addition to these benefits, many vegetables are high in the EFAs and contain special nutrients that are tremendously beneficial to the human body.

Do not have more than two alcoholic beverages per week. If you have a couple (two) glasses of alcohol per week, it should have no effect. Your body will absorb it, and you won't even see it. Any greater alcohol consumption becomes a ball and chain wrapped around your waist that you drag with you 24 hours a day. The alcoholic portion of any beverage you consume *will* be converted to body-fat. For women, this body-fat is gathered at the back of the arms, the hips and just below the belly button. For men, it seems to gather between the chest and the pelvic area.

The correct supplementation program can dramatically enhance your results. My experience with thousands of clients has proven that the proper diet combined with a well-designed supplementation program will provide an average of approximately *30% increased rate of fat reduction*. In addition to faster and greater fat reduction, you can achieve a stronger immune system, higher energy levels, and most important, a higher success rate of maintenance. You will find a comprehensive guide to these supplements in Chapter 5.

Meal replacement "Protein bars" are an excellent way to have a meal in a hurry or on-the-go. Depending on which plan you have chosen, you will be required to eat 4–7 times per day. In many cases, this is a difficult task, one that can be made much easier with the option of having a meal replacement bar. Just open the wrapper and eat your meal—it is as easy as that. You can use these bars as often as needed, as long as they contain the appropriate amounts of proteins, carbohydrates and fats. There are many of these bars available. The trick is to find the bar that contains the necessary amounts of proteins, carbohydrates, and fats for your plan. To find the right bar, just go to your local health food store and either look at the labels yourself, or ask for help. You can also call (888) 663-2881 to have some of the right bars sent to you.

It's simple. You are ready. You'll do great!

## 10

THE HI/LO PLAN

EASE

I won't paint any rosy pictures for you. This is a difficult program to follow and you will crave carbohydrates from time to time. You must be willing to sacrifice for 2 to 3 weeks.

EATING OUT

Because of the strict guidelines of food choices and portion sizes, this is not any easy plan to follow when you are at a restaurant. It can be done, but I strongly recommend that you do not eat out for at least the first week, so you can better gauge the demands of the program.

RATE OF FAT LOSS

While this is one of the most difficult programs to follow, it has great potential in terms of your fat-loss payoff. The results you will achieve while on this plan will definitely be dramatic. I have seen women lose as much as 18 pounds of body-fat in three weeks. I have seen men lose 16 pounds of body-fat in three weeks. The average three-week loss will be 10 pounds of body-fat for women and 8 pounds of body-fat for men.

ENERGY LEVEL

Unlike most all of the other nutritional programs in this book, you may not feel like you are at peak performance levels while on this plan. This program will make you feel good most of the time, but there will be instances when you feel your energy lag. The Hi/Lo is not a long-term health plan, it's about losing body-fat today.

DURATION

The Hi/Lo is definitely a temporary plan. It is not a long-term way of eating. The 21-day plan should be done an absolute maximum of two times in succession. The 14-day version should never be done more than three times in succession. In between each cycle, you should take three or four days off, to let your body recover. If, after completing two or three cycles of the Hi/Lo, you wish to go on it again, you must allow one month of eating in a less aggressive manner. When finished with the program you should revisit the "Is This You?" questions to determine what you should do next.

The Hi/Lo is based on the serious and intensive manipulation of the metabolism. This manipulation will enable the body to use stored fat as its primary energy source. The Hi/Lo is based on metabolic trickery, that occurs by bringing the body close to starvation, and bringing it back out of starvation by giving it food. By keeping the body uncomfortably close to starvation, it allows the most possible fat to be liberated or eliminated from the body without loss of energy.

The Hi/Lo will not work for everyone, but it does work for the majority. The people it does work for, it works very, very well. This program is for the person who has large quantities of fat to lose, and not a lot of time to do so. This plan requires sacrifice, but there is a big payoff in store for you if you have the discipline to stick to this program 100%.

In most diet chapters contained in this book, I have given an overview of what may be occurring within your hormonal balance, or more to the point, the lack of balance associated with the hormones.

By choosing this nutritional program, you have come to this particular chapter based on situational needs and goals surrounding the need for speedy and significant fat reduction. In more cases than not, you have gotten to this point because of hormonal imbalances, and the Hi/Lo will indeed be effective in this respect. Through an atomic bomb–like approach, this program brings instantaneous harmony between insulin, glucagon, cortisol, and growth hormone. The Hi/Lo is not a plan that will fix any of your hormonal problems permanently; it just brings temporary balance. These hormonal buttons are being pushed very hard on this plan, and while it brings instantaneous benefit, it must be mentioned that this program has the potential to do harm to your metabolism if you repeat this diet more times than I have suggested. If you decide to do this plan more than the suggested duration, you are taking that responsibility into your own hands. It is certainly my recommendation that you do not exceed the time-frame guidelines for this diet.

The Hi/Lo has very specific food choices. It is important that you eat *only* those foods listed—*there are no substitutions*. The plan also calls for very specific amounts of these foods and it is very important to eat *only those amounts*. There is a short list of foods that are free foods. These foods can be eaten at any time, in any amount, as many times a day as you like. This list is very limited and should not be varied from. When you stick to this program 100% you will be *very* pleased with your results.

On the Hi/Lo Plan, you will eat four meals per day, separated by no more than four hours. On each day, for each meal, you will have a portion of protein, and a portion of carbohydrates or vegetables. The portions of carbohydrates and vegetables will be different, depending on whether you are on a "Hi" or "Lo" cycle. Everything should be cooked as cleanly as possible, using little, or no fat.

The Hi/Lo plan is separated into cycles. The Hi cycle provides an intake of starchy carbohydrates, which is followed by a Lo cycle where the carbohydrate allowance comes from vegetables, or a very low-carbohydrate day. You may choose the 14- or 21-day plan. The

14-day schedule begins with two days of Lo, followed by two days of Hi, repeating this cycle until day 9. Days 9–14 are all Lo days. The 21-day plan alternates two days of Lo followed by two days of Hi, until day 17. Days 17–21 are all Lo days. The 5-day low cycle, which ends either plan, will usually yield twice the fat-loss as that of the previous days, and you will definitely be amazed by what you see in the mirror.

THE HI/LO SCHEDULE

The 14-day version

1. Lo day	6. Lo day	11. Lo day
2. Lo day	7. Hi day	12. Lo day
3. Hi day	8. Hi day	13. Lo day
4. Hi day	9. Hi day	14. Lo day
5. Lo day	10. Lo day	

The 21-day version

1. Lo day	8. Hi day	15. Hi day
2. Lo day	9. Lo day	16. Hi day
3. Hi day	10. Lo day	17. Hi day
4. Hi day	11. Hi day	18. Lo day
5. Lo day	12. Hi day	19. Lo day
6. Lo day	13. Lo day	20. Lo day
7. Hi day	14. Lo day	21. Lo day

HERE'S HOW YOU DO IT

First you must determine your portion sizes:

Women who weigh 150 pounds or less

20 • Have 28 grams of protein per meal (Hi or Lo meals)
10 • Have 15 grams of carbohydrates per Hi meal
10 • Have 10 grams of vegetable carbohydrates per Lo meal

Women who weigh more than 150 pounds

- Have 35 grams of protein per meal (Hi or Lo meals)
- Have 20 grams of carbohydrates per Hi meal
- Have 15 grams of vegetable carbohydrates per Lo meal

Men who weigh 170 pounds or less

- Have 40 grams of protein per meal (Hi or Lo meals)
- Have 25 grams of carbohydrates per Hi meal
- Have 20 grams of vegetable carbohydrates per Lo meal

Men who weigh more than 170 pounds

- Have 50 grams of protein per meal (Hi or Lo meals)
- Have 35 grams of carbohydrates per Hi meal
- Have 25 grams of vegetable carbohydrates per Lo meal

Now that you know your portion sizes, go to the food lists and fill in the blanks. Simply take the number of grams of protein you need to have each meal and calculate your portions. Then insert the number into the space provided.

If you have determined that you need 28 grams of protein, you take 28 and divide it by the number of grams of protein in an ounce of chicken breast, which is 7. You would then need to eat 4 ounces of chicken breast per serving.

If you need to have 15 grams of vegetable carbohydrates per meal on Lo days, simply take that number and divide it by the amount of vegetable carbohydrates in a cup of broccoli, which is 10. You would have 1.5 cups of broccoli.

THE LO AND THE HI MEALS

You will begin with two Lo days. On the Lo days, you take one selection from each group (proteins and vegetables) four times per day. You may have half the amount of one item and half of another or mix and match any way you wish—just get the equivalent to one portion from each group, four times per day.

Then you'll have two Hi days. On the Hi days, your first two meals will consist of one portion of protein and one portion of carbohydrate. Choose one food from each group (proteins and carbohydrates). Again, you may mix and match, as long as you consume the equivalent to one portion. The last two meals on Hi days will consist of one portion of protein and one portion of vegetables (no carbohydrates).

You may have the "Free Foods" at any time in any amount, with or without meals.

After two Hi days, you repeat the cycle. You will always be alternating two Lo, two Hi, two Lo, two High, etc., until the end of the plan, when you'll complete several Lo days in succession.

After you have completed the 14- or 21-day cycle, you will have two options:

1. Take five days off, and repeat the cycle. If you choose to do this, you will need a plan to follow while waiting to restart the Hi/Lo. Choose *any* one of the other plans in this book (except the one-week quick fix). *You must take at least five days off before beginning a successive cycle of the Hi/Lo.*
2. Revisit the "Is This You?" questions and find the appropriate plan to follow next.

WHAT TO EXPECT

The Hi/Lo works very well, but you will have to work at it to get the best results. Your first two days, which are Lo days, will be very difficult. You will be hungry, you will crave sugars and carbohydrates. Your energy will not be at its best. Your body will need these two days to begin the metabolic processes that the Hi/Lo promotes.

The next 7 days (14-day plan) or 14 days (21-day plan) will be easier than the first two days, but still an effort. The foods are not everyday foods that will be readily available. You will need to eat at home most of the time, and when you do eat out, you will need to pay very close attention to what you are eating. Make sure it is the right stuff.

The last 5 days, which are all Lo days, will be the most difficult, but will have the great benefit. You will be low on energy, hungry, grumpy, crave sweets, and you will be very tired of the foods you have been eating. Endure the struggle and you will be happy you did.

Table 10.01

Hi/Lo Plan Food List (Lo Days)

Proteins

(All four meals)

All proteins to be prepared fat-free

__3__ oz. Chicken breast (7 grams of protein per oz.)

__3__ oz. Turkey breast (7 grams of protein per oz.)

__3__ oz. Fish/Shellfish (7 grams of protein per oz.)

__7__ Egg whites (3 grams of protein each)

__20__ Protein powder (Check # of grams of protein per scoop)

Microfiltered, ion-exchanged, predigested whey is best.

Lo day vegetables

(All four meals)

All vegetables to be prepared fat-free

__1__ Cup(s) Broccoli (equal to 10 carbohydrates per cup)

__1__ Cup(s) Green beans (equal to 10 carbohydrates per cup)

__1__ Cup(s) Bell peppers (equal to 10 carbohydrates per cup)

__1__ Cup(s) Squash/Zucchini (equal to 10 carbohydrates per cup)

__1__ Cup(s) Cauliflower (equal to 10 carbohydrates per cup)

__1__ # of Asparagus spears (equal to 1 carbohydrate each)

Table 10.02

Hi/Lo Plan Food List (Hi Days)

Proteins

(All four meals)

All proteins to be prepared fat-free

_____ oz. Chicken breast (7 grams of protein per oz.)

_____ oz. Turkey breast (7 grams of protein per oz.)

_____ oz. Fish/Shellfish (7 grams of protein per oz.)

__6__ Egg whites (3 grams of protein each)

_____ Protein powder (Check # of grams of protein per scoop)

Microfiltered, ion-exchanged, predigested whey is best.

Hi day carbohydrates

(First two meals)

All carbohydrates to be prepared fat-free

__1/4__ Cup(s) Oats (measure dry) (50 carbohydrates per cup)

__1½__ oz. Red potato (7 grams carbohydrates per oz.)

__1½__ oz. Yams/Sweet potato (7 grams carbohydrates per oz.)

_____ Brown rice (35 grams carbohydrate per oz.)

__⅓ c__ Beans/Legumes (38 carbohydrates per cup)

Hi day vegetables

(Last two meals)

All vegetables to be prepared fat-free

_____ Cup(s) Broccoli (equal to 10 carbohydrates per cup)

_____ Cup(s) Green beans (equal to 10 carbohydrates per cup)

_____ Cup(s) Bell peppers (equal to 10 carbohydrates per cup)

_____ Cup(s) Squash/Zucchini (equal to 10 carbohydrates per cup)

_____ Cup(s) Cauliflower (equal to 10 carbohydrates per cup)

_____ # of Asparagus spears (equal to 1 carbohydrate each)

Table 10.03

Free Foods for the Hi/Lo Plan

Vinegar	Diet beverages
Lemon juice	Decaffeinated coffee
Lime juice	Sparkling water
Mustard	Water
Garlic	Iced tea
Mushrooms	Herbal tea
Onions	Dry seasonings (Herbal, etc.)
Scallions	Salt
Cucumber	Pepper
Lettuce	Sugar-free Jell-O
Citrus peels	Sugar-free gum
Chili peppers	

HELPFUL HINTS

It is absolutely essential that you drink plenty of water while on the Hi/Lo Plan. The more water you can consume, the faster you will be eliminating fat from your body. You should get in the habit of carrying a bottle of water around with you. You should be certain to consume at least ten 8-oz. glasses of water per day. It would be far preferable to drink at least two 64-oz. bottles of water per day. If you drink a can of diet soda, or have a glass of iced tea, this will count as one glass of water.

You must not miss meals. If you do not eat **four** times a day you will not succeed. For this more than any other plan, **preparation is key.** Know that if you will be in the middle of nowhere when mealtime rolls around, that you will have brought something to eat with you. If you know that you will be in the middle of a meeting when mealtime comes around, bring a meal replacement in with you, so that you do not activate your starvation-protection mechanism. You don't have to eat a meal, you just have to ingest the proper amounts of carbohydrate, protein and fat. Prepare a thermos full of protein drink, to have throughout the day. Don't go out into the world everyday, and just expect that the right food will be there. It won't be there. Think ahead. Plan for your success.

Weigh and measure everything you eat. Do not assume it is the right amount. Do not guess the amount of any of the portions. Get it right and reap the benefits. If you are unable to locate a food scale, you may call toll-free (888) 663–2881.

Stay cool. Keeping the air temperature around you lower than usual can help to accelerate the speed at which you can lose fat. Your body will be forced to burn more calories to maintain normal body temperature. 80% of the extra calories will come straight from your fat stores. (This trick stops working after about one month.)

If you happen to overeat one meal, do not *undereat during the next meal*. In other words, do not alter any meal, based on a mistake you made on the meal prior to that, or in anticipation of a meal that is ahead of you. By doing this you will have ruined *two* meals. Each meal is its own separate entity, and is not reliant on any other meal. Each meal is like taking a medicine that we are trying to get an effect from, that will wear off in a few hours, so we would take that medicine again. If you change the medicine once, would you change the medicine again to account for that? No. You can't double up, you can't cut it in half. You will simply be ruining a half of your day instead of a quarter of a day. Even in cases of extreme overeating, the next meal is exactly as it should be. We are attempting to create an environment for your metabolism. Allow that environment to be as stable as possible. The same applies to undereating. Do not eat more the next time.

Make sure you are getting enough protein. Most menu items will not have the necessary protein content. You must learn to order additional portions, or let them know exactly how much you need. You must make an Olympian effort to get enough protein.

Foods must be eaten together, at the same time, to bring about the desired results. A major point of eating in this prescribed manner is to stimulate or repress the production of specific hormones that make up the metabolism. To foster this hormone activity, these foods must be ingested as a whole. Do not, under any circumstances, have a protein without the carbohydrate/vegetable portion of the meal or vice versa. These food groups will always be consumed at the same time, or eating will have the exact opposite outcome than the results you desire.

Do not have more than two alcoholic beverages per week. If you have a couple (two) glasses of alcohol per week, it should have no effect. Your body will absorb it, and you won't even see it. Any greater alcohol consumption and it is a ball and chain wrapped around your waist that you are dragging with you 24 hours a day. The alcoholic portion of any beverage you consume WILL be converted to body-fat. For women this body-fat is gathered at the back of the arms, the hips and just below the belly button. For men, it seems to gather between the chest and the pelvic area.

Do at least 45 minutes of cardiovascular exercise, at least three times per week. Read the chapter about exercise to determine how to design your exercise program. Do two weight-training sessions per week, one for the upper body and one for the lower body.

The correct supplementation program can dramatically enhance your results. My experience with thousands of clients has proven that the proper diet combined with a well-designed supplementation program will provide an average of approximately *30% increased rate of fat reduction*. In addition to faster and greater fat reduction, you can achieve a stronger immune system, higher energy levels, and most importantly a higher success rate of maintenance. You will find a comprehensive guide to these supplements in Chapter 5.

Meal replacement "Protein bars" are an excellent way to have a meal in a hurry or on-the-go. Depending on which plan you have chosen, you will be required to eat 4–7 times per day. In many cases, this is a difficult task, one that can be made much easier with the option of having a meal replacement bar. Just open the wrapper and eat your meal—it is as easy as that. You can use these bars as often as needed, as long as they contain the appropriate amounts of proteins, carbohydrates, and fats. There are many of these bars available. The trick is to find the bar that contains the necessary amounts of proteins, carbohydrates and fats for your plan. To find the right bar, just go to your local health food store and either look at the labels yourself, or ask for help. You can also call (888) 663-2881 to have some of the right bars sent to you.

## 11

THE 50/30/20 PLAN

EASE

Because of the high amount of carbohydrates and the smaller amount of protein, you should find this plan to be very easy to follow. You should find the types of foods you need just about anywhere.

EATING OUT

While you are on this plan, every restaurant, every fast food outlet, every grocery store will have something you can eat.

RATE OF FAT LOSS

People who are fortunate enough to be on this program will lose fat easily. This is not an aggressive attack on fat, rather this plan is for people with a gifted metabolism who are trying to find a way of eating that is best suited for their needs. If this diet is truly right for you, you probably do not have a large amount of fat to lose. If this is the case, you should expect to lose 1–3 pounds of body-fat per week.

ENERGY LEVEL

Your energy level should be at an all-time high while you are eating this way. No more mid-afternoon slumps, no more "I can't get out of bed." You should feel better from the get-go and stay stable from there.

DURATION

If this diet applies to you, you will find that it will always apply to you. You can and should remain on this type of eating program for the rest of your life. Yours is not the type of metabolism that needs temporary fixing. You are looking for a permanent solution. You should start eating in this way now, and continue eating this way forever.

If at any time along the way you begin to feel that your body is not responding the same, just re-visit the "Is This You?" questions and find what you'll do to rebalance.

YOUR UNIQUE METABOLISM

Your answers to the "Is This You?" questions indicate that you are among a small handful of lucky people who have somehow escaped the hazards of the modern-day diet. Your answers show that you are not experiencing metabolic pandemonium, as most readers of this book are, and so you won't have any significant hurdles to clear in attaining your goals. You should have a fairly easy time of reducing your level of body-fat and gaining vitality. You should, by balancing your diet as I will suggest within this chapter, make rapid progress. Statistically, persons who fit your profile have fewer incidences of heart disease, diabetes, strokes, obesity, and high cholesterol. This is due to the fact that your "big four" hormones (see Chapter 2) are well balanced. It is usually when these hormones become imbalanced that the above mentioned maladies strike. You may be asking, "If I am so gifted, why am I still fat?" The answer is very simple. You have never been taught the way to eat that best suits your unique metabolism. You have never eaten foods that your body requires. You need only make small changes to your daily diet and begin to enjoy big changes in your appearance and the way you feel.

The 50/30/20 is my choice for a person like you. This plan will fine tune your body and get it working better than ever before. There should be no need for you to change to any other plan, because with your metabolism working as well as it does now, coupled with improvements this plan will cause, you should attain all your goals and then maintain them easily. You will probably stay on this plan forever.

Now let's get going!

THE PLAN

This plan requires you to consume **four** equally balanced and equally spaced meals per day. You should have breakfast, lunch, a mid-afternoon meal, and dinner. The food choices on this plan are widely available and popular foods that you will be able to find almost anywhere. Your meals will be made up of 50% carbohydrate, 30% protein, and 20% fat. There is also a lengthy list of foods that are "free foods." In between, during, and in addition to the four meals you must eat per day, you may draw from this list of "free" foods any time you desire.

The prescribed ratio of 50% carbohydrate, 30% protein, and 20% fat is the type of meal that we, as Americans, have been led to perceive as a "balanced" meal. In truth, this is not a balanced diet at all. It is very high in carbohydrates. Your diet is designed in this way because your particular metabolism requires a larger percentage of carbohydrates, and a moderate intake of protein and fat.

This plan allows you a lot of freedom, in that, there are a wide range of food choices that will be available most anyplace you may be. You will not have to shop at health-food stores or eat out of boxes. Unless you want to.

75% of the gifted metabolisms that find their way to this chapter are simply *eating too little*. The other 25% of you lucky people are divided up between those that are eating too much, too seldom, eating too frequently, eating unbalanced meals, too much at one time, or eating right before bedtime.

What you will accomplish in eating balanced meals at regular intervals will be to achieve a significantly higher energy level that will stay at that level, and last throughout the day until just before bedtime. You will also see improvements in your skin and hair quality. Your thought process will be much clearer. Creativity will return. The fogginess that is undoubtedly in your head now will leave, and a crisp and clear thought process will replace it. Short-term and long-term memory will vastly improve. Your bowel movements will improve. The frequency of urination for most people will go up to about ten times per day. This is a very good thing, as you will be voiding that unwanted body-fat in the process. You will also eliminate sugar and chocolate cravings, or the strange eating binges you may be experiencing. These cravings, which are probably your downfall, will subside immediately because you are "filling in the blanks" with food that your body needs. You will be processing these new food choices, and the proper amount of those foods in a very efficient manner. You will become a walking meal clock, in that, hunger will be present only just before mealtime. You will wake up hungry in the morning, and you should eat breakfast before you leave the house. (Unless, of course, you are leaving the house to eat breakfast.)

After you determine the proper amounts of food that makes the perfect meal for you, you will be hungry every three to five hours. This will eliminate your need for the instant energy gratification that sweets have afforded you in the past. You will not even have to think about what time it is. After two or three days, you will know what time it is by your level of hunger.

YOUR BODY'S ENERGY (CALORIE) REQUIREMENTS

The first step in getting started on your new plan will be to determine the approximate number of calories to consume each meal. The necessary formulas appear on the following pages. It really is not complicated. In fact, it is very simple to complete these calculations. You should use the book like a workbook—write on the pages, fill in the blanks.

Basal Energy Requirement (BER)

The first step in designing your personal nutritional program is to determine your basal energy requirement (BER). The BER is the amount of energy your body requires in order to fuel its most basic functions. The BER is the approximate number of calories needed to breathe, think, pump blood through veins, etc.

There will be two different formulas for the BER. One for those who have had their body-fat measured, and one for those who have not. Once again, it is highly recommended that you have your bodyfat measured prior to starting your nutritional plan. The BER is much more accurately determined if you know your fat percentage. If you have not had your fat measured, skip this section and proceed to the next.

The first step in determining the BER is to determine the amount of lean body weight you have. As we discussed in Chapter 1, lean body weight is the amount of your body that is not fat. It is the portion of your body that is composed of muscle, organs, bones, water, and other nonfat tissues.

For those who know their body-fat percentage, the formula to determine the amount of lean body weight is as follows. If you have not had your body-fat measured, skip this and go to the next section.

Body weight _____ × Body-fat% _____ = Fat weight _____

Body weight _____ – Fat weight _____ = **Lean body weight (LBW)** _____

Example

A person who weighs 100 lbs. with a body-fat of 15% will have 15 pounds of fat. This person would then have 85 lbs. of lean body weight (100 - 15 = 85). Once you have determined your lean body weight (LBW), the next step is to factor in your age.

Age Factor

Now take your lean body weight (LBW) and **multipy it by your age factor**. You will then have your basal energy requirement (BER).

- 50 years or older, the age factor is 13
- 40–50 years, the age factor is 14
- 20–40 years, the age factor is 15
- Up to 20 years, the age factor is 16

For example, a person with a LBW of 100 lbs., who is 36 years old, will have a BER of 1500. (100 × 15 = 1500)

Now, calculate your own BER.

LBW _____ × Age factor _____ = BER _____

Total Energy Requirement (TER)

Remember—the BER is the approximate number of calories your body will require to do nothing but exist. If you are active, you will need to adjust the BER to account for the energy expended during the activities. This number will be your total energy requirement or your TER. The total energy requirement (TER) is the approximate number of calories that your body will require to keep itself alive, *and* to perform the various activities of the day. In order to determine your TER, you will need to factor in your level of activity.

Activity Factor

The activity factor is used to approximate the number of calories you will need to consume to replace the amount of energy expended during exercise and other activities. Take your BER and add the appropriate number from the list below. If you are not active, skip this calculation.

- If you participate in up to 30 minutes of exercise/activity per day, multiply your LBW by 2.

- If you participate in 30–60 minutes of exercise/activity per day, multiply your LBW by 3.
- If you participate in 60–90 minutes of exercise/activity per day, multiply your LBW by 4.

Example

A person who has a BER of 1500 calories and a lean body weight of 100 lbs., who exercises 60 minutes per day (activity factor = LBW multiplied by 3) will end up with a number of 1800. BER 1500 + ACTIVITY FACTOR 300 = 1800. This number is the TER, or total energy requirement.

Now calculate your own activity factor.

LBW = _____ × (2, 3, or 4) _____ = activity factor _____

Now determine your total energy requirement (TER).

BER = _____ + activity factor _____ = TER _____

(If you are inactive, your BER is the same as your TER.)

Adjusted Total Energy Requirement (AFTER)

Remember—the TER is the approximate number of calories you would consume in a day if you wanted to maintain your current status. However, if you want to lose some body-fat, you will need to give your body a reason to use the fat as fuel. With few exceptions, this is accomplished by reducing the caloric intake to well below what your body requires to do the day's work. This adjusted calorie amount is known as the adjusted total energy requirement (ATER). As long as all the hormones are doing their jobs, and your metabolism is in a state of balance, the significant deficit of energy will cause your body to go into its fat reserves to get the missing energy. Hence, a reduction in body-fat.

To calculate your adjusted total energy requirement (ATER), simply take your TER and subtract 500.

Example

TER 1800 - 500 = 1300. (1300 is the ATER)

Now calculate your own adjusted total energy requirement (ATER).

TER _____ −500 = _____ ATER

This number reflects the approximate number of calories you need to consume each day while attempting to lose body-fat. When you have lost all the fat you want to lose, use your TER as your daily caloric intake.

ENERGY (CALORIE) REQUIREMENTS WITHOUT A BODY-FAT MEASUREMENT

Caution: These formulas are only 70% accurate without a measurement of your body-fat percentage. *I recommend that you have your body-fat measured as soon as possible.*

Estimated Total Energy Requirement (ETER)

The estimated total energy requirement (ETER) is the approximate amount of energy (calories) that your body will need in a day to perform its basic functions (such as breathing and thinking), *in addition to* what it will require to complete the usual amount of exercise/activity.

Use the following guide to determine your ETER.

STEP ONE IS TO MULTIPLY YOUR BODY WEIGHT BY YOUR WEIGHT FACTOR.

Weight Factor

The weight factor is an approximation of the total amount of energy (calories) that a person of your weight, with an average amount of body-fat would need in a day just to maintain normal body function, such as breathing, thinking, etc. Use the following list to determine your weight factor.

- **Women** who weigh up to 120 lbs.—multiply your weight by *8.5*
- **Women** who weigh between 121 and 150 lbs.—multiply your weight by *8.25*
- **Women** who weigh between 151 and 200 lbs.—multiply your weight by *8*
- **Women** who weigh between 200 and 250 lbs.—multiply your weight by 7
- **Women** who weigh more than 250 lbs.—multiply your weight by *6.5*
- **Men** who weigh up to 165 lbs.—multiply your weight by *10*
- **Men** who weigh 166 and 190 lbs.—multiply your weight by *9.5*
- **Men** who weigh more than 190 lbs.—multiply your weight by *9.25*

Now calculate your own weight factor.

Body weight _____ × _____ (weight factor) = _____

STEP TWO IS TO APPLY YOUR ACTIVITY FACTOR.

Activity Factor

The activity factor is used to approximate the number of calories you will need to consume to replace the amount of energy expended during exercise and other activities. Take your weight factor and add the appropriate number from the list below. If you are sedentary, skip this calculation.

- If you participate in up to 30 minutes of exercise/activity per day, add .5 calories per pound of body weight to your weight factor
- If you participate in 30–60 minutes of exercise/activity per day, add 1 calorie per pound of body weight to your weight factor
- If you participate in more than 60 minutes of exercise/activity per day, add 1.5 calories per pound of body weight to your weight factor

Example

A male who weighs 176 lbs. has a weight factor of 1672 (176 × 9.5 = 1672).

If he exercises 60 minutes per day, he has an activity factor of 176 (1 cal. × 176 lbs. = 176).

So, his estimated total energy requirement (ETER) would be 1848 (1672 + 176 = 1848).

Now, calculate your own ETER.

Weight factor _____ + activity factor _____ = *ETER* _____

YOUR IDEAL 50/30/20 MEAL

Now that you have successfully determined how many calories you will need each day, you'll need to break that down into calories per meal. You will also need to determine where you are going to get those calories from. You must calculate the grams of carbohydrates, proteins and fats per meal. The formulas required to accomplish these calculations are simple—let's take a look.

Begin by taking your adjusted total energy requirement (ATER) or your estimated total energy requirement (ETER) and dividing it by 4. This number will be calories per meal.

ATER or ETER _____ ÷ 4 = _____ Calories per meal

Now that you have determined the approximate number of calories to consume each meal, you'll have to break that down to grams of carbohydrate, protein, and fat per meal.

Take the number of calories each of the three meals will have, and multiply it by 50%, 30%, and 20% (carbohydrate, protein, and fat).

Calories per meal _____ × 50% = _____ Carbohydrate calories per meal

Now, because carbohydrate contains 4 calories per gram, divide the above number by 4 to determine the number of *grams* of carbohydrate per meal.

Carbohydrate calories per meal _____ ÷ 4 = _____ **Grams of carbohydrate per meal**

Now you'll need to calculate the protein portion of each meal. Take the number of calories per meal and multiply it by 30%.

Calories per meal _____ ÷ 30% = _____ Calories from protein for each meal

Because protein contains 4 calories per gram, divide the above number by 4 to determine the number of grams of protein per meal.

Protein calories per meal _____ ÷ 4 = _____ **Grams of protein per meal**

Now use the same formula to determine the fat content of each meal. Take the number of calories per meal and multiply it by 20%.

Calories per meal _____ ÷ 20% = _____ Fat calories per meal

Now, because fat contains 9 calories per gram, take the number of fat calories per meal and divide it by 9—this will be the number of fat grams per meal.

Fat calories per meal _____ ÷ 9 = _____ **Grams of fat per meal**

Now let's summarize the figures.

- **Grams of carbohydrate per meal** _____
- **Grams of protein per meal** _____
- **Grams of fat per meal** _____

PUTTING THE NUMBERS TO WORK

Now that you have successfully completed all the necessary calculations for the plan, it's time to put them into action. Getting the right amounts of the different food groups is very important, so take your time and make sure you fully understand. You may need to read this part of the chapter two times, but once you really understand all these numbers, you will be equipped to have great success.

Portion Sizes

Determining your portion sizes is fairly easy, it just takes a couple of simple steps. Simply take the number of grams of carbohydrate, protein, or fat you need per meal, and divide it by the number of grams of carbohydrate per portion listed on the food list.

Example #1

Let's say that you need 21 grams of protein per meal. You have chosen to have chicken breast. Chicken breast contains 7 grams of protein per oz., so you would have 3 oz. (21 grams protein ÷ 7 grams Protein/Oz. = 3 oz.).

Example #2

If you needed 40 grams of carbohydrate per meal, and you chose to eat rice, you would have about one cup, because *cooked* rice contains about 37 grams carbohydrate per cup (40 grams carbohydrate ÷ 37 grams carbohydrate in a cup = about one cup).

All amounts listed on the food list are after cooking, except oatmeal, which is measured prior to cooking. I highly recommend that you weigh your portions a few times to become familiar with what amounts you should be eating. After just a few times weighing these foods, you will be able to "eyeball" the amounts.

If you do not see a particular food that you want to eat on the list, avoid the food for the first month. After that, simply determine how much carbohydrate, protein and fat the food contains, and calculate how much you need to have. Remember, though—avoid all non-listed foods for the first month.

Table 11.01

50/30/20/ Plan Food List

PROTEINS

Chicken breast*

Turkey breast*

Venison*

Beefalo*

Buffalo*

Fish*

Shellfish*

Lamb

Veal

7% fat ground beef

Lean steaks

Lean cuts of pork

Canadian bacon

Ham
Average 7 grams protein/oz.

Egg whites*
3 grams protein each

Egg substitute*
Check label for protein content.

Nonfat cottage cheese *Average 3 grams protein/oz.*

Nonfat cheese
Average 9 grams protein/oz.

Tofu/Soy protein products
Check label for protein content. Watch for extra carbs and fats.

Protein powders*
*Microfiltered, ion-exchanged, predigested **whey** protein is best.*

CARBOHYDRATES

Yams/Sweet potatoes*

Red potatoes*
7 grams carbohydrate/oz.

Rice*
37 grams carbohydrate/cup

Oats*
27 grams carbohydrate ½ cup—uncooked

Beans/Lentils*
Average 35 grams carbohydrate/cup

Breads
Check label for carbohydrate content.

Bagels
Average 50 carbohydrates per bagel—check label.

Corn tortillas
Average 12 carbohydrates each

Flour tortillas
Average 20 carbohydrates each—check label.

Fruit
Average 35 carbohydrates per small piece

Melon
Average 45 carbohydrates per melon

Pasta
38 carbohydrates per cup

FATS

Safflower oil*

Sunflower oil*

Hemp oil*

Olive oil*

Canola oil*

Peanut oil*

Tahini oil*

Soybean oil*
Best not to cook oils 4 grams fat per tsp.

Nuts*
Check label for fat content.

Nut butters*
Average 3 grams fat per tsp.

Avocado*
3 grams fat per tbsp.

Olives*
1 gram fat each

Seeds*
Average 12 grams fat/oz.

Butter
9 grams fat per pat 14 grams fat per tbsp.

Mayonnaise
14 grams fat per tbsp.

Cream
5 grams fat per tbsp.

Cheese
Check label for fat content.

*Indicates best choices
All amounts listed are after cooking

Table 11.02

Free Foods List

The following foods are free foods. Unless otherwise noted, you can consume them at any time, with or without meals.

All vegetables *Except corn, peas, squash, carrots, beets*
Diet sodas *Avoid those containing phosphoric acid or caffeine or saccharin*
Diet flavored waters *Avoid those containing phosphoric acid or caffeine or saccharin*
Crystal Light
Regular coffee *Up to 2 cups per day*
Unlimited decaffeinated coffee *Preferably water processed*
Herbal teas *Caffeine-free*
Iced tea *Sugar-free; avoid saccharin; decaffeinated; green tea is best*
Swiss Miss diet cocoa *Up to 2 packets per day*
Sugar-free Jell-o
Sugar-free gum
Frozen yogurt *Maximum 4 oz., 2 times per week*
Gise Frozen Yogurt (800) 448-4473
Nonfat sour cream
Nonfat cream cheese
Nonfat mayonnaise
Nonfat salad dressing *Maximum of 2 tbsp. per day*
Citrus peels
Vinegars
Lemon and lime juice
Extracts
All dry seasonings and herbal seasonings
**BBQ, Teriyaki, Mustard, Relish, Salsa, Ketchup, A-1,
Soy sauce (low sodium)**

Note: Consumption of aspartame-containing food products is a personal decision. Much data exists to support its safety, but this continues to be a much-debated issue.

YOUR FIRST WEEK

It is an understatement to say that during your first week your body will be going through significant changes. You will be bringing back balance to what may have been unbalanced for your entire life. You may have never in your life arrived at what is correct for you. Because you are reading this book, you probably haven't. During this first week, you will be rearranging the metabolism. As a result, you may be feeling certain things that are unusual for you. You may be depressed, or you may feel euphoric. You may get some acne, or you may eliminate the acne that you have. Your energy may soar, keeping you up at night, or you may feel totally lethargic for the first week. You will go through a number of metabolic changes that will result in symptoms that I am not able to predict.

What you must do is keep moving forward, no matter what. No matter how you feel. I liken this to the way you would drive a car. You place your foot on the gas pedal, and the car begins to move forward. If you hold the gas pedal down, the car travels faster and faster. As the car travels faster, it also uses up more fuel. This fuel consumption allows the car to travel even faster. What happens when you let your foot off the gas pedal? The car slows back down. In other words, if you deprive yourself of food, you will not have enough gas in your engine. If you feel like you are eating too much, or change the way you should be eating because you are feeling a certain way, *you will **never** get over the hump*. You will never reach freeway speeds, and you will be stuck on side-streets forever. So keep going forward no matter what. For this first week you will have to go on faith. Don't let up, and you will be well on your journey.

HELPFUL HINTS

You must not miss meals. If you do not eat **four** times a day at least 80% of the time, you will not succeed.

If you happen to overeat one meal, do not undereat during the next meal. In other words, do not alter any meal, based on a mistake you made on the meal prior to that, or in anticipation of a meal that is ahead of you. By doing this you will have ruined *two* meals. Each meal is its own separate entity, and is not reliant on any other meal. Each meal is like taking a medicine that we are trying to get an effect from, that will wear off in a few hours, so we would take that medicine again. If you change the medicine once, would you change the medicine again to account for that? No. You can't double up, you can't cut it in half. You will simply be ruining a half of your day instead of a quarter of a day. Even in cases of extreme overeating, the next meal is exactly as it should be. We are attempting to create an environment for your metabolism. Allow that environment to be as stable as possible. The same applies to undereating. Do not eat more the next time.

You've heard it a hundred times, but I'll say it again. You must drink enough water. If you are dehydrated, you will not burn fat. End of story. Water is necessary in the process of not only fat reduction, but every metabolic process. If you are not drinking enough water, you will fail. You should be urinating about ten times per day for your fat to remove itself from your body. If you are not in the bathroom more than you think you should be, you are not in there enough. Drink at least eight 12-oz. glasses of water each day.

Another suggestion I would make would be to purchase a food scale. Don't assume that you know anything, even if you have been on a program where you had to weigh your food. It is vital that you are getting the proper amount of food in the correct ratios for this to work for you. You don't want to be, and you don't need to be measuring everything that you eat. However, for the first week or so, I want you to get a better idea of what your portion size will look like. If you have determined, by using "The Perfect Portion," that you need 6 oz. of protein with each meal, weigh that out before and after cooking. Put it in your bowl of salad or on the plate, so that you can be accustomed to what that portion size looks like. Give yourself that edge, you'll thank me for it down the road. If you are unable to locate a scale, call toll-free (888) 663–2881.

For this or any other plan, preparation is key. Know that if you will be in the middle of nowhere when mealtime rolls around, you will have brought something to eat with you. If you know that you will be in the middle of a meeting when mealtime comes around, bring a meal replacement in with you, so that you do not activate your starvation-protection mechanism. You don't have to eat a meal, you just have to ingest the proper amounts of carbohydrate, protein, and fat. Prepare a thermos full of a meal replacement drink, to have throughout the day. Don't go out into the world everyday, and just expect that the right food will be there. It won't be there. Think ahead. Plan for your success.

Make sure you are getting enough protein. Most menu items will not have the necessary protein content. You must learn to order additional portions, or let them know exactly how much you need. You must make an Olympian effort to get enough protein.

Foods must be eaten together at the same time to bring about the desired results. A major point of eating in this prescribed manner is to stimulate or repress the production of specific hormones that make up the metabolism. To foster this hormone activity, these foods must be ingested as a whole. Do not, under any circumstances, have a protein without the fat portion of the meal or vice versa. These food groups will always be consumed at the same time, or eating will have the exact opposite outcome than the results you desire.

Do not have more than two alcoholic beverages per week. If you have a couple (two) glasses of alcohol per week, it should have no effect. Your body will absorb it, and you won't even see it. Any greater alcohol consumption and it is a ball and chain wrapped around your waist that you are dragging with you 24 hours a day. The alcoholic portion of any beverage you consume *will* be converted to body-fat. For women this body-fat is gathered at the back of the arms, the hips and just below the belly button. For men, it seems to gather between the chest and the pelvic area.

The correct supplementation program can dramatically enhance your results. My experience with thousands of clients has proven that the proper diet combined with a well-designed supplementation program will provide an average of approximately *30% increased rate of fat reduction*. In addition to faster and greater fat reduction, you can achieve a stronger immune system, higher energy levels, and most importantly a higher success rate of maintenance. You will find a comprehensive guide to these supplements in Chapter 5.

Meal replacement "Protein bars" are an excellent way to have a meal in a hurry or on-the-go. Depending on which plan you have chosen, you will be required to eat 4–7 times per day. In many cases, this is a difficult task, one that can be made much easier with the option of having a meal replacement bar. Just open the wrapper and eat your meal—it is as easy as that. You can use these bars as often as needed, as long as they contain the appropriate amounts of proteins, carbohydrates and fats. There are many of these bars available. The trick is to find the bar that contains the necessary amounts of proteins, carbohydrates, and fats for your plan. To find the right bar, just go to your local health food store and either look at the labels yourself, or ask for help. You can also call (888) 663-2881 to have some of the right bars sent to you.

Are you ready to get started? You're going to do great!

## 12

THE 7-DAY QUICK FIX

EASE

*T*his plan is not easy to follow, and is definitely not for the weak of heart. This plan is for the person that is willing to give up just about everything for a week in an effort to lose some body-fat in a hurry.

EATING OUT

It will be nearly impossible for you to eat out while on this plan. I recommend that you either eat at home or take your meals with you each day.

RATE OF FAT LOSS

This plan usually works extremely well. I have seen people lose 10 pounds of fat in one week. The average result is 6 pounds (of fat).

ENERGY

You will probably feel very well the majority of the time. There will be times when your energy will be less than optimal, but the plan lasts only one week.

DURATION

You will be on this plan for seven days and seven days only. If you choose to repeat this program, you must wait at least 4 weeks. At the end of the week you should consult the "Is This You?" portion of the book to choose a more appropriate plan.

THE PLAN

You did not choose this plan based on your metabolism. You chose this plan because you have a deadline by which you must look better than you do now. You are pressured by this deadline, and you are willing to make sacrifices to make your grand appearance at some event that is about a week from today. Does that sound about right?

It is a very rare occasion when I recommend this nutritional program for a client. This is not my first or even my second choice, but it is a very effective choice for clients that have an appearance, photo shoot, or special event, that requires that they look their leanest. I will assume that you have an upcoming wedding, prom, or some special event to attend, and you feel that you need to be much thinner in one week. For you, I can only say that your prayers have been answered.

This plan requires unflinching discipline and dedication. The good news is that you need only maintain this high level of restriction for one week. *Only stay on this diet for one week!* After seven days, the results will diminish drastically. If you were really foolish, and stayed on this diet longer than the duration I recommend, you would begin to see that any results you had achieved would reverse, and in fact, you would get fatter with each day. This plan is to be used for 7 days and 7 days only. Commit to this program 100%, do exactly what I recommend, nothing more and nothing less, and in only one week you will have up to 10 pounds less fat than you have today. Any less than 95% commitment and the results won't be worth the sacrifice.

This diet is definitely the exception to the rule, compared with other diets outlined in this book. Where the other nutritional programs would be similar to a cross-country trip on the freeway, this particular diet is more like a drag race. Where your body will need at least one week to adjust to the food combinations outlined in the other nutritional programs, this diet will begin to start working with your first meal. This plan is a very aggressive attack on fat, and will not reward you with the positive health benefits that all the other plans in this book do. In fact, this plan can become a detriment to your energy and wellness if you exceed the prescribed 7 days.

The 7-Day Quick Fix is very simple. You eat exactly what is detailed on the menu for your weight category. There are no substitutions or adjustments. You will eat 5 meals per day, all five of which are predetermined. There are no choices. On this plan you will not need to determine your need for calories or portion sizes. Very simply, your sex and your desired body weight will be the only factors involved in this equation. Your body weight will determine how much food you will need each day that you are on this program.

This plan has four different alternatives: Women with a body weight of less than 126 pounds, women with a body weight of more than 125 pounds, men with a body weight of over 175 pounds, and men with a body weight of less than 176 pounds. Figure out how much you weigh, and follow the plan that fits your profile. After you have read the plan, make sure to finish the chapter—there will be very valuable information that will apply to everyone while they are on this nutritional program. This additional information will enhance your results by at least 50%. After you read and re-read this chapter, do your grocery shopping, and get ready to lose some fat. *Here we go.*

Table 12.01

Women with a Body Weight of Less Than 126 Lbs.

You will have five meals per day, and eat every three hours.

Your first four meals

The first four meals of each day will be exactly the same. You will have:

1 protein shake
providing 20 grams of protein

This protein shake should be made from predigested, ion-exchanged, microfiltered whey.

½ of a grapefruit
10 raisins
3 capsules of "Total EFA"

Your fifth meal

Eaten no later than 2½ hours before bedtime, this meal will consist of a portion of protein, a small amount of vegetables, and a portion of good clean fat.

PROTEIN CHOICES (Choose one)
3 oz. (after cooking) of chicken breast,
turkey breast, fish, or 7 egg whites

You may mix and match proteins as long as you have the equivalent to one portion.

1 cup of
VEGETABLES
No squash, carrots, peas, beets, corn, or broccoli
FAT CHOICES (Choose one)
1 teaspoon of olive oil, or flax oil, or safflower oil
Or
4 almonds, or 4 walnuts, or ⅛ avocado, or 5 olives

Table 12.02

Women with a Body Weight of More Than 125 Lbs.

You will have five meals per day, and eat every three hours.

Your first four meals

The first four meals of each day will be exactly the same. You will have:

1 protein shake
providing 28 grams of protein

This protein shake should be made from predigested, ion-exchanged, microfiltered whey.

½ of a grapefruit
10 raisins
3 capsules of "Total EFA"

Your fifth meal

Eaten no later than 2½ hours before bedtime, this meal will consist of a portion of protein, a small amount of vegetables, and a portion of good clean fat.

PROTEIN CHOICES (Choose one)
5 oz. (after cooking) of chicken breast,
turkey breast, fish, or 12 egg whites

You may mix and match proteins as long as you have the equivalent to one portion.

1.5 cup of
VEGETABLES
No squash, carrots, peas, beets, corn, or broccoli
FAT CHOICES (Choose one)
1 teaspoon of olive oil, or flax oil, or safflower oil
Or
4 almonds, or 4 walnuts, or ⅛ avocado, or 5 olives

Table 12.03

Men with a Body Weight of Less Than 176 Lbs.

You will have five meals per day, and eat every three hours.

Your first four meals

The first four meals of each day will be exactly the same. You will have:

1 protein shake
providing 38 grams of protein

This protein shake should be made from predigested, ion-exchanged, microfiltered whey.

1¼ of a grapefruit
20 raisins
5 capsules of "Total EFA"

Your fifth meal

Eaten no later than 2½ hours before bedtime, this meal will consist of a portion of protein, a small amount of vegetables, and a portion of good clean fat.

PROTEIN CHOICES (Choose one)
6 oz. (after cooking) of chicken breast,
turkey breast, fish, or 16 egg whites

You may mix and match proteins as long as you have the equivalent to one portion.

1.5 cup of
VEGETABLES
No squash, carrots, peas, beets, corn, or broccoli
FAT CHOICES (Choose one)
2 teaspoons of olive oil, or flax oil, or safflower oil
Or
9 almonds, or 9 walnuts, or ³⁄₈ avocado, or 12 olives

Table 12.04

Men with a Body Weight of More Than 175 lbs.

You will have five meals per day, and eat every three hours.

Your first four meals

The first four meals of each day will be exactly the same. You will have:

1 protein shake
providing 45 grams of protein

This protein shake should be made from predigested, ion-exchanged, microfiltered whey.

1 ¼ grapefruit
23 raisins
5 capsules of "Total EFA"

Your fifth meal

Eaten no later than 2½ hours before bedtime, this meal will consist of a portion of protein, a small amount of vegetables, and a portion of good clean fat.

PROTEIN CHOICES (Choose one)
8 oz. (after cooking) of chicken breast,
turkey breast, fish, or 18 egg whites

You may mix and match proteins as long as you have the equivalent to one portion.

2 cups of
VEGETABLES
No squash, carrots, peas, beets, corn, or broccoli
FAT CHOICES (Choose One)
2 teaspoons of olive oil, or flax oil, or safflower oil
Or
9 almonds, or 9 walnuts, or ³/₈ avocado, or 12 olives

Free Foods for the 7-Day Quick Fix

Vinegar	Diet beverages
Lemon juice	Decaffeinated coffee
Lime juice	Sparkling water
Mustard	Water
Garlic	Iced tea
Mushrooms	Herbal tea
Onions	Dry seasonings (Herbal, etc.)
Scallions	Salt
Cucumber	Pepper
Lettuce	Sugar-free Jell-O
Citrus peels	Sugar-free gum
Chili peppers	

THERE ARE 5 RULES YOU MUST FOLLOW WHILE ON THIS PLAN

These are not helpful hints, rather they are a *must* for those of you who have chosen this plan. As you have only a week, these additional rules will push the body's buttons very hard, and you will double your results by adding these keys of success.

You must drink 128 oz. of water per day (1 gallon). This may seem like an overwhelming amount of liquid, but it will flush the fat by-products and rapidly accumulating toxins from your body each and every time you eliminate that water. 128 oz. is equal to one gallon. This could be sixteen 8-oz. glasses or two 64-oz. bottles (the tall ones) that you would buy at the store. My suggestion would be to fill a gallon jug, and take it with you everywhere. Any caffeine-free, water-based beverage counts as water.

You must do at least 60 minutes of cardiovascular exercise each and every day. It would be optimal if you could do two 60-minute sessions, one in the morning and one in the early evening. You should also do some variation of weight training. You may refer to Chapter 4 for examples. Note: On any other plan, it is not necessary or very productive to do this much exercise.

If possible, you should take a steam or sauna bath once a day for the next week (check with your physician first). This will eliminate any extra water from under your skin, and also help to detoxify your body, as the skin is the largest eliminative system in the body.

Get full body sun exposure at least three times during this week. You should absorb the rays of the sun for 10–20 minutes on three different occasions. If weather or climate prohibits you from doing this, you may choose to lay in a tanning bed for 10–15 minutes three times this week. This will dry the skin, drawing all that water you will be drinking out from every pore. Believe me, it will greatly enhance your results, and the little color you get will make you look all the better. **Please note:** This is an insignificant amount of UV exposure.

You must get at least eight hours of sleep per night. You will be driving you body very hard this week. If your body is not rested you will drive it into an over-trained and undernourished state. If this happens, you will significantly decrease the results you would have enjoyed. Rest. It is one of the keys to your success.

HELPFUL HINTS

Preparation is key for this or any plan. Go to the store and get everything you will need over the next week. Do it now. It is going to be very easy to prepare the first four meals, but you are going to have to take it to work. Make sure that you have it with you on the road, and haul it around with you. After you get home from the grocery store, you may even consider separating it into portions, and putting it in containers.

Weigh and measure everything you eat. Do not assume it is the right amount. Do not guess the amount of any of the portions. Get it right and reap the benefits.

Stay cool. Keeping the air temperature around you lower than usual can help to accelerate the speed at which you can lose fat. Your body will be forced to burn more calories to maintain normal body temperature. 80% of the extra calories will come straight from your fat stores. (This trick only works for about a month.)

The correct supplementation program can dramatically enhance your results. My experience with thousands of clients has proven that the proper diet combined with a well-designed supplementation program will provide an average of approximately *30% increased rate of fat reduction*. In addition to faster and greater fat reduction, you can achieve a stronger immune system, higher energy levels, and most importantly a higher success rate of maintenance. You will find a comprehensive guide to these supplements in Chapter 5.

## 13

THE 30/50/20 PLAN

EASE

*T*his plan is relatively easy to follow, in that you will be able to eat normal everyday foods. This is a high protein moderate carbohydrate, low fat approach to reduce body-fat. Because the balance between these food groups is weighted heavily on the protein side, you will need to make some adjustments to insure you get the proper percentages.

EATING OUT

Eating out is fairly easy. Just about any restaurant will have the food that you need. The foods that are on your plan are everyday food, however they will not be everyday amounts. To accommodate these amounts, you will have to learn how to order, make special requests, and let your desired portion sizes be known so that you may get what you need to succeed.

RATE OF FAT LOSS

Compared to everything you have tried in the past, your fat loss on this nutritional plan will be rapid. You should expect to lose 2–4 pounds of body-fat per week.

ENERGY

Your energy will go up immediately, and remain absolutely stable. You will never again experience the ups and downs in you energy during the day, and may in fact, feel more vital than you have ever felt.

DURATION

This is not a long-term plan, and there soon will come a time when you need to move onto another nutritional program. You will know when it is time to do this, because the results that you have had will suddenly cease, and you will reach a plateau. You will be doing everything that you have been doing, your results will be very steady, you will feel great, you will have followed the program closely, and then for three or four weeks you will not get those same results. To get to this point will take anywhere from two months to a year. Your goal on this plan is to reach that plateau. When this is achieved, it will mean that the hormonal imbalance that is now present will have been corrected. It is then time to revisit the "Is This You?" questions, and discover what to do next.

YOUR UNIQUE METABOLISM

Now that you have found your way to the 30/50/20, take a moment to learn a little bit about your unique metabolism. Based on your answers to the "Is This You?" questions, it seems that your body has become very carbohydrate-sensitive and as a result of this, the hormones that make up your metabolism have become unbalanced.

Although it appears that your problems are not severe, they are significant. You are experiencing symptoms that are consistent with the beginning stages of hyperinsulinemia, or excessive secretion of insulin, as well as symptoms that indicate elevations of cortisol and glucagon. It will be literally impossible for you to reduce the amount of fat in your body without eliminating these problems. The problems you have are common. Your body will however, require some unusual tactics to repair itself. The good news is that these problems can and will be eliminated by the 30/50/20 over time.

This nutritional program will help you to eliminate these problems by:

1. Significantly reducing the amount of sugars/carbohydrates in your diet, which will help to lower insulin levels.
2. The small but consistent intake of carbohydrates will help to regulate glucagon.
3. The frequent feeding and high-protein intake will help to lower cortisol levels.
4. The specific 30/50/20 ratio will stabilize glucose, allowing your body to gain control over appetite, cravings, and hormones.

Once you have gained control over the sugar in your blood and the hormones that make up your metabolism, you will experience much greater energy, no cravings, better sleep, sharper thinking, stronger muscles, more endurance, and of course—*fat loss*.

The 30/50/20 is "just what the doctor ordered" for your situation. It is the plan of all plans for you right now. When you follow the 30/50/20 you will see that food is the most powerful medicine on earth.

I have designed this plan specifically for the types of imbalances that you are currently facing. Use this tool wisely and gain piece of mind and wellness that you have never before experienced.

Now, let's get started!

THE PLAN

The 30/50/20 is a high-protein, low-carbohydrate, low-fat nutritional plan. You will be required to consume four equally balanced and spaced meals each and every day. Ideally, these four meals should be spaced about four hours apart. You should have breakfast, lunch, a mid-afternoon meal, and dinner. The food choices on this plan are widely available and popular foods that you will be able to find almost anywhere. The meals that you eat will be made up of 30% carbohydrate, 50% protein, and 20% fat. There is also a lengthy list of foods that are "free" foods. In between, during, and in addition to the four meals you must eat per day, you may draw on this list of "free" foods any time you desire. You may have these foods in any amount as often as you like, at any time you like.

The prescribed ratio of 30% carbohydrate, 50% protein, and 20% fat is truly a balanced meal for your current metabolic state. Your diet is designed in this way because your particular metabolism requires the high energy afforded by eating a larger percentage of protein in relation to carbohydrates and fat. This plan allows you a lot of freedom, in that there are a wide range of food choices. You will not be limited to eating out of a box, or having to shop at a specialty health food store for groceries.

What you will accomplish in eating balanced meals at regular intervals will be to achieve a significantly higher energy level that will stay at that level, and last throughout the day until an hour or so before bedtime. You will also see improvements in your skin and hair quality. Your thought process will be much clearer. Creativity will return. The fogginess that is undoubtedly in your head now will leave, and a crisp and clear thought process will replace it. Short-term and long-term memory will vastly improve. Your bowel movements will improve. The frequency of urination for most people will go up to about ten times per day. This is a very good thing, as you will be voiding that unwanted body-fat in the process.

By eating a balanced meal at regular intervals, you will be effectively balancing all the hormones that are at work when you eat. The most significant change will be the additional protein you will be eating. For you the perfect meal may be an entirely new concept that may include some new foods. You will be processing these new food choices, and the proper amount of those foods at a very efficient rate. You will become a walking meal clock, in that, hunger will be present only just before mealtime. You will not even have to think about what time it is. After two or three days, you will know what time it is by your level of hunger. You will wake up hungry in the morning, and you should eat breakfast before you leave the house. (Unless, of course, you are leaving the house to eat breakfast.) After you determine the proper amounts of food that makes the perfect meal for you, you will be hungry every three to five hours. This will eliminate your need for the instant energy gratification that sweets have afforded you in the past.

The first step in designing your own personal version of the 30/50/20 is to calculate the approximate amount of food you'll be eating each meal. The necessary formulas appear on the following pages. Take some time to complete them. I recommend that you write in the book, use it as a workbook.

DETERMINING YOUR BODY'S ENERGY (CALORIE) REQUIREMENTS

Basal Energy Requirement (BER)

The first step in designing your personal nutritional program is to determine your basal energy requirement (BER). The BER is the amount of energy your body requires in order to fuel its most basic functions. The BER is the approximate number of calories needed to breathe, think, pump blood through veins, and so on.

There will be two different formulas for the BER. One for those who have had their body-fat measured, and one for those who have not. Once again, it is highly recommended that you have your body-fat measured prior to starting your nutritional plan.

The BER is much more accurately determined if you know your fat percentage. If you have not had your fat measured, skip this section and proceed to the next.

The first step in determining the BER is to determine the amount of lean body weight you have. As we discussed in Chapter 1, lean body weight is the amount of your body that is not fat. It is the portion of your body that is composed of muscle, organs, bones, water, and other nonfat tissues.

For those who know their body-fat percentage, the formula to determine the amount of lean body weight is as follows. If you have not had your body-fat measured, skip this and go to the next section.

Body weight _____ × Body-fat% _____ = Fat weight _____

Body weight _____ – Fat weight _____ = Lean body weight
(LBW) _____

Example

A person who weighs 100 lbs. with a body-fat of 15% will have
15 pounds of fat. This person would then have 85 lbs. Of lean body
weight (100 – 15 = 85). Once you have determined your lean body
weight (LBW), the next step is to factor in your age.

Age Factor

Now take your lean body weight (LBW) and *multiple it by your
age factor.* You will then have your basal energy requirement (BER).

- 50 years or older, the age factor is 13
- 40–50 years, the age factor is 14
- 20–40 years, the age factor is 15
- Up to 20 years, the age factor is 16

For example, a person with a LBW of 100 lbs., who is 36 years
old, will have a BER of 1500. (100 × 15 = 1500)
Now, calculate your own BER.

LBW _____ × Age factor _____ = BER _____

Total Energy Requirement (TER)

Remember—the BER is the approximate number of calories your body will require to do nothing but exist. If you are active, you will need to adjust the BER to account for the energy expended during the activities. This number will be your total energy requirement or your TER. The total energy requirement (TER) is the approximate number of calories that your body will require to keep itself alive, *and* to perform the various activities of the day. In order to determine your TER, you will need to factor in your level of activity.

Activity Factor

The activity factor is used to approximate the number of calories you will need to consume to replace the amount of energy expended during exercise and other activities. Take your BER and add the appropriate number from the list below. If you are not active, skip this calculation.

- If you participate in up to 30 minutes of exercise/activity per day, multiply your LBW by 2.
- If you participate in 30–60 minutes of exercise/activity per day, multiply your LBW by 3.
- If you participate in 60–90 minutes of exercise/activity per day, multiply your LBW by 4.

Example

A person who has a BER of 1500 calories and a lean body weight of 100 lbs., who exercises 60 minutes per day (activity factor = LBW multiplied by 3) will end up with a number of 1800. BER 1500 + ACTIVITY FACTOR 300 = 1800. This number is the TER, or total energy requirement.

Now calculate your own activity factor.

LBW = _____ × (2, 3, or 4) _____ = Activity factor _____

Now determine your total energy requirement (TER)

BER = _____ + Activity factor _____ = TER _____

(If you are inactive, your BER is the same as your TER.)

Adjusted Total Energy Requirement (ATER)

Remember—the TER is the approximate number of calories you would consume in a day if you wanted to maintain your current status. However, if you want to lose some body-fat, you will need to give your body a reason to use the fat as fuel. With few exceptions, this is accomplished by reducing the caloric intake to well below what your body requires to do the day's work. This adjusted calorie amount is known as the adjusted total energy requirement (ATER). As long as all the hormones are doing their jobs, and your metabolism is in a state of balance, the significant deficit of energy will cause your body to go into its fat reserves to get the missing energy. Hence, a reduction in body-fat.

To calculate your adjusted total energy requirement (ATER), simply take your TER and subtract 500.

Example

TER 1800 × 500 = 1300. (1300 is the ATER)
Now calculate your own adjusted total energy requirement (ATER).

TER _____ – 500 = _____ ATER

This number reflects the approximate number of calories you need to consume each day while trying to reduce your level of body-fat.

DETERMINING YOUR BODY'S ENERGY (CALORIE) REQUIREMENTS WITHOUT A BODY-FAT MEASUREMENT

Caution: These formulas are only 70% accurate without a measurement of your body-fat percentage. *I recommend that you have your body-fat measured as soon as possible.*

Estimated Total Energy Requirement (ETER)

The estimated total energy requirement (ETER) is the approximate amount of energy (calories) that your body will need in a day to perform its basic functions (such as breathing and thinking), ***in addition to*** what it will require to complete the usual amount of exercise/activity.

Use the following guide to determine your ETER.

STEP ONE IS TO MULTIPLY YOUR BODY WEIGHT BY YOUR WEIGHT FACTOR.

Weight Factor

The weight factor is an approximation of the total amount of energy (calories) that a person of your weight, with an average amount of body-fat would need in a day just to maintain normal body function, such as breathing, thinking, etc. Use the following list to determine your weight factor.

- **Women** who weigh up to 120 lbs.—multiply your weight by *8.5*
- **Women** who weigh between 121 and 150 lbs.—multiply your weight by *8.25*
- **Women** who weigh between 151 and 200 lbs.—multiply your weight by *8*
- **Women** who weigh between 200 and 250 lbs.—multiply your weight by *7*
- **Women** who weigh more than 250 lbs.—multiply your weight by *6.5*
- **Men** who weigh up to 165 lbs.—multiply your weight by *10*
- **Men** who weigh 166 and 190 lbs.—multiply your weight by *9.5*

- **Men** who weigh more than 190 lbs.—multiply your weight by *9.25*

Now calculate your own weight factor.

Body weight _____ × _____ (weight factor) = _____

STEP TWO IS TO APPLY YOUR ACTIVITY FACTOR.

Activity Factor

The activity factor is used to approximate the number of calories you will need to consume to replace the amount of energy expended during exercise and other activities. Take your weight factor and add the appropriate number from the list below. If you are sedentary, skip this calculation.

- If you participate in up to 30 minutes of exercise/activity per day, add .5 calories per pound of body weight to your weight factor
- If you participate in 30–60 minutes of exercise/activity per day, add 1 calorie per pound of body weight to your weight factor
- If you participate in more than 60 minutes of exercise/activity per day, add 1.5 calories per pound of body weight to your weight factor

Example

A male who weighs 176 lbs. has a weight factor of 1672. (176 × 9.5 = 1672)

If he exercises 60 minutes per day, he has an activity factor of 176. (1 cal × 176 lbs.=176)

So, his *Estimated* total energy requirement (ETER) would be 1848. (1672 + 176 = 1848)

Now, calculate your own ETER.

Weight factor _____ + activity factor _____ = ETER _____

YOUR IDEAL 30/50/20 MEAL

Now that you have determined your ATER or ETER, you'll need to divide the total number of calories between your four daily meals, and divide the calories per meal into grams of carbohydrate, protein, and fat. The calculations you'll use to accomplish this are very simple. Ready? Good. Let's do it.

Begin by taking your adjusted total energy requirement (ATER) or your estimated total energy requirement (ETER) and dividing it by 4. This number will be calories per meal.

ATER or ETER _____ ÷ 4 = _____ Calories per meal

Now that you have determined the approximate number of calories to consume each meal, you'll have to break that down to grams of carbohydrate, protein, and fat per meal.

Take the number of calories each of the three meals will have, and multiply it by 30%, 50%, and 20%.

Calories per meal _____ × 30% = _____ Carbohydrate calories per meal

Now, because carbohydrate contains 4 calories per gram, divide the above number by 4 to determine the number of *grams* of carbohydrate per meal.

Carbohydrate calories per meal _____ ÷ 4 = _____ **Grams of carbohydrate per meal**

Now you'll need to calculate the protein portion of each meal. Take the number of calories per meal and multiply it by 50%.

Calories per meal _____ × 50% = _____ Calories from protein for each meal

Because protein contains 4 calories per gram, divide the above number by 4 to determine the number of grams of protein per meal.

Protein calories per meal _____ ÷ 4 = _____ **Grams of protein per meal**

Now use the same formula to determine the fat content of each meal. Take the number of calories per meal and multiply it by 20%.

Calories per meal _____ × 20% = _____ Fat calories per meal

Now, because fat contains 9 calories per gram, take the number of fat calories per meal and divide it by 9—this will be the number of fat grams per meal.

Fat calories per meal _____ ÷ 9 = _____ **Grams of fat per meal**

Now let's summarize the figures.

- **Grams of carbohydrate per meal** _____
- **Grams of protein per meal** _____
- **Grams of fat per meal** _____

PUTTING THE NUMBERS TO WORK

Now that you have successfully completed all the necessary calculations for the plan, its time to put them into action. Getting the right amounts of the different food groups is very important, so take your time and make sure you fully understand. You may need to read this part of the chapter two times, but once you really understand all these numbers, you will be equipped to have great success.

Portion Sizes

Determining your portion sizes is fairly easy, it just takes a couple of simple steps. Simply take the number of grams of carbohydrate, protein, or fat you need per meal, and divide it by the number of grams of carbohydrate per portion listed on the food list.

Example #1

Let's say that you need 21 grams of protein per meal. You have chosen to have chicken breast. Chicken breast contains 7 grams of protein per oz., so you would have 3 oz. (21 grams protein ÷ 7 grams protein/oz. = 3 oz.).

Example #2

If you needed 40 grams of carbohydrate per meal, and you chose to eat rice, you would have about one cup, because *cooked* rice contains about 37 grams carbohydrate per cup. (40 grams carbohydrate ÷ 37 grams carbohydrate in a cup = about one cup.)

All amounts listed on the food list are after cooking, except oatmeal, which is measured prior to cooking. I highly recommend that you weigh your portions a few times to become familiar with what amounts you should be eating. After just a few times weighing these foods, you will be able to "eyeball" the amounts.

If you do not see a particular food that you want to eat on the list, avoid the food for the first month. After that, simply determine how much carbohydrate, protein and fat the food contains, and calculate how much you need to have. Remember, though—avoid all non-listed foods for the first month.

Table 13.01

30/50/20/ Plan Food List

PROTEINS

Chicken breast*
Turkey breast*
Venison*
Beefalo*
Buffalo*
Fish*
Shellfish*
Lamb
Veal
7% fat ground beef
Lean steaks
Lean cuts of pork
Canadian bacon
Ham
Average 7 grams protein/oz.

Egg whites*
3 grams protein each

Egg substitute*
Check label for protein content.

Nonfat cottage
cheese *Average 3 grams protein/oz.*

Nonfat cheese
Average 9 grams protein/oz.

Tofu/Soy protein
products
Check label for protein content. Watch for extra carbs and fats.

Protein powders*
Microfiltered, ion-exchanged, predigested **whey** *protein is best.*

CARBOHYDRATES

Yams/Sweet pota-
toes*

Red potatoes*
7 grams carbohydrate/oz.

Rice*
37 grams carbohydrate/cup

Oats*
27 grams carbohydrate 1/2 cup—uncooked

Beans/Lentils*
Average 35 grams carbohydrate/cup

Breads
Check label for carbohydrate content.

Bagels
Average 50 carbohydrates per bagel—check label.

Corn tortillas
Average 12 carbohydrates each

Flour tortillas
Average 20 carbohydrates each—check label.

Fruit
Average 35 carbohydrates per small piece

Melon
Average 45 carbohydrates per melon

Pasta
38 carbohydrates per cup

FATS

Safflower oil*
Sunflower oil*
Hemp oil*
Olive oil*
Canola oil*
Peanut oil*
Tahini oil*
Soybean oil*
Best not to cook oils 4 grams fat per tsp.

Nuts*
Check label for fat content.

Nut butters*
Average 3 grams fat per tsp.

Avocado*
3 grams fat per tbsp.

Olives*
1 gram fat each

Seeds*
Average 12 grams fat/oz.

Butter
9 grams fat per pat 14 grams fat per tbsp.

Mayonnaise
14 grams fat per tbsp.

Cream
5 grams fat per tbsp.

Cheese
Check label for fat content.

*Indicates best choices
All amounts listed are after cooking

Table 13.02

Free Foods List

The following foods are free foods. Unless otherwise noted, you can consume them at any time, with or without meals.

All vegetables *Except corn, peas, squash, carrots, beets*
Diet sodas *Avoid those containing phosphoric acid or caffeine or saccharin*
Diet flavored waters *Avoid those containing phosphoric acid or caffeine or saccharin*
Crystal Light
Regular coffee *Up to 2 cups per day*
Unlimited decaffeinated coffee *Preferably water processed*
Herbal teas *Caffeine-free*
Iced tea *Sugar-free; avoid saccharin; decaffeinated; green tea is best*
Swiss Miss diet cocoa *Up to 2 packets per day*
Sugar-free Jell-o
Sugar-free gum
Frozen yogurt *Maximum 4 oz., 2 times per week*
Gise Frozen Yogurt (800) 448-4473
Nonfat sour cream
Nonfat cream cheese
Nonfat mayonnaise
Nonfat salad dressing *Maximum of 2 tbsp. per day*
Citrus peels
Vinegars
Lemon and lime juice
Extracts
All dry seasonings and herbal seasonings
BBQ, Teriyaki, Mustard, Relish, Salsa, Ketchup, A-1,
Soy sauce (low sodium)

Note: Consumption of aspartame-containing food products is a personal decision. Much data exists to support its safety, but this continues to be a much-debated issue.

YOUR FIRST WEEK

It is an understatement to say that during your first week your body will be going through significant changes. You will be bringing back balance to what may have been unbalanced for your entire life. You may have never in your life arrived at what is correct for you. Because you are reading this book, you probably haven't. During this first week, you will be rearranging the metabolism. As a result, you may be feeling certain things that are unusual for you. You may be depressed, or you may feel euphoric. You may get some acne, or you may eliminate the acne that you have. Your energy may soar, keeping you up at night, or you may feel totally lethargic for the first week. You will go through a number of metabolic changes that will result in symptoms that I am not able to predict.

What you must do is keep moving forward, no matter how what. No matter how you feel. I liken this to the way you would drive a car. You place your foot on the gas pedal, and the car begins to move forward. If you hold the gas pedal down, the car travels faster and faster. As the car travels faster, it also uses up more fuel. This fuel consumption allows the car to travel even faster. What happens when you let your foot off the gas pedal? The car slows back down. In other words, if you deprive yourself of food, you will not have enough gas in your engine. If you feel like you are eating too much, or change the way you should be eating because you are feeling a certain way, *you will* ***never*** *get over the hump*. You will never reach freeway speeds, and you will be stuck on side-streets forever. So keep going forward no matter what. For this first week you will have to go on faith. Don't let up, and you will be well on your journey.

HELPFUL HINTS

You must not miss meals. If you do not eat **four** times a day at least 80% of the time, you will not succeed.

If you happen to overeat one meal, do **not** ***undereat during the next meal***. In other words, do not alter any meal, based on a mistake you made on the meal prior to that, or in anticipation of a meal that is ahead of you. By doing this you will have ruined *two* meals. Each meal is its own separate entity, and is not reliant on any other meal. Each meal is like taking a medicine that we are trying to get an effect from, that will wear off in a few hours, so we would take that medicine again. If you change the medicine once, would you change the medicine again to account for that? No. You can't double up, you can't cut it in half. You will simply be ruining a half of your day instead of a quarter of a day. Even in cases of extreme overeating, the next meal is exactly as it should be. We are attempting to create an environment for your metabolism. Allow that environment to be as stable as possible. The same applies to undereating. Do not eat more the next time.

You've heard it a hundred times, but I'll say it again. You must drink enough water. If you are dehydrated, you will not burn fat. End of story. Water is necessary in the process of not only fat reduction, but every metabolic process. If you are not drinking enough water, you will fail. You should be urinating about ten times per day for your fat to remove itself from your body. If you are not in the bathroom more than you think you should be, you are not in there enough. Drink at least eight 12-oz. glasses of water each day.

Another suggestion I would make would be to purchase a food scale. Don't assume that you know anything, even if you have been on a program where you had to weigh your food. It is vital that you are getting the proper amount of food in the correct ratios for this to work for you. You don't want to be, and you don't need to be measuring everything that you eat. However, for the first week or so, I want you to get a better idea of what your portion size will look like. If you have determined, by using "The Perfect Portion," that you need 6 oz. of protein with each meal, weigh that out before and after cooking. Put it in your bowl of salad or on the plate, so that you can be accustomed to what that portion size looks like. Give yourself that edge, you'll thank me for it down the road. If you are unable to locate a scale, call toll-free (888) 663–2881.

For this or any other plan, preparation is key. Know that if you will be in the middle of nowhere when mealtime rolls around, you will have brought something to eat with you. If you know that you will be in the middle of a meeting when mealtime comes around, bring a meal replacement in with you, so that you do not activate your starvation-protection mechanism. You don't have to eat a meal, you just have to ingest the proper amounts of carbohydrate, protein, and fat. Prepare a thermos full of a meal replacement drink, to have throughout the day. Don't go out into the world everyday, and just expect that the right food will be there. It won't be there. Think ahead. Plan for your success.

Make sure you are getting enough protein. Most menu items will not have the necessary protein content. You must learn to order additional portions, or let them know exactly how much you need. You must make an Olympian effort to get enough protein.

Foods must be eaten together at the same time to bring about the desired results. A major point of eating in this prescribed manner is to stimulate or repress the production of specific hormones that make up the metabolism. To foster this hormone activity, these foods must be ingested as a whole. Do not, under any circumstances, have a protein without the fat portion of the meal or vice versa. These food groups will always be consumed at the same time, or eating will have the exact opposite outcome than the results you desire.

It is most beneficial to have vegetables with each meal. Vegetables will not only eliminate any trace of carbohydrate craving, but will also be very filling, and regulate the bowels very successfully. In addition to these benefits, many vegetables are high in the EFAs and contain special nutrients that are tremendously beneficial to the human body.

Do not have more than two alcoholic beverages per week. If you have a couple (two) glasses of alcohol per week, it should have no effect. Your body will absorb it, and you won't even see it. Any greater alcohol consumption and it is a ball and chain wrapped around your waist that you are dragging with you 24 hours a day. The alcoholic portion of any beverage you consume *will* be converted to body-fat. For women this body-fat is gathered at the back of the arms, the hips and just below the belly button. For men, it seems to gather between the chest and the pelvic area.

The correct supplementation program can dramatically enhance your results. My experience with thousands of clients has proven that the proper diet combined with a well-designed supplementation program will provide an average of approximately *30% increased rate of fat reduction*. In addition to faster and greater fat reduction, you can achieve a stronger immune system, higher energy levels, and most importantly a higher success rate of maintenance. You will find a comprehensive guide to these supplements in Chapter 5.

Meal replacement "Protein bars" are an excellent way to have a meal in a hurry or on-the-go. Depending on which plan you have chosen, you will be required to eat 4–7 times per day. In many cases, this is a difficult task, one that can be made much easier with the option of having a meal replacement bar. Just open the wrapper and eat your meal—it is as easy as that. You can use these bars as often as needed, as long as they contain the appropriate amounts of proteins, carbohydrates and fats. There are many of these bars available. The trick is to find the bar that contains the necessary amounts of proteins, carbohydrates, and fats for your plan. To find the right bar, just go to your local health food store and either look at the labels yourself, or ask for help. You can also call (888) 663-2881 to have some of the right bars sent to you.

Are you ready to get started?
I'm positive you are. Let's go!

## 14

THE 3+2 PLAN

EASE

*T*his is an extremely easy program to follow. The program is very accommodating, and is not a "strict" diet in any sense. The plan allows for three meals that are similar to what you may be already eating, with the addition of two protein intensive snack-like meals.

EATING OUT

The selection of foods, along with the balance between the food groups makes it a very easy plan to stick to when eating out. This is about as easy as it gets.

RATE OF FAT LOSS

The rate of fat loss while on this plan will be significant, especially for a person who is metabolically challenged. Certainly the rate of loss will be proportionate with the level of effort required to adhere to the plan. Typical results will be 2–4 pounds of *fat loss* per week.

ENERGY LEVEL

While following this plan your energy levels will remain high and consistent. You should have none of the usual mid-afternoon slumps, peaks and valleys, etc. You will wake up clear and feel tired only just before bedtime.

DURATION

By answering "yes" to the majority of "Is This You?" questions, you have indicated that this plan will work exceptionally well for your body. You very well may choose to adhere to the plan for the rest of your life. One could and should stay on this program for as long is it is effective, however, you may want to revisit the "Is This You?" questions after a few months to determine if a different plan will work better for your newly redesigned metabolism.

The 3+2 is a nutritional program that I have designed for people *just like you*.

THIS PLAN REQUIRES 3 MEALS PER DAY AND 2 PROTEIN SNACKS

The 3+2 program will allow you to change the characteristics of your metabolism that have sabotaged your progress in the past. Utilizing the 3+2 plan will enable you to shed the unwanted body-fat and inches. This nutritional program will also *increase* your energy level while *decreasing* your risk of many diseases. These results will be permanent because you will correct the very hormonal imbalances that are at the heart of your problems. These hormones are intimately involved in the process of fat loss and must be balanced for any long-term success to take place. It is important to know that you are not doing something temporary here. While you are worried about the here and now, and would like to look and feel better today, it is of much greater concern what will happen tomorrow and next year. The 3+2 plan will not only get you through today and tomorrow but will help to insure that you stay thin and healthy for the long term.

YOUR UNIQUE METABOLISM

Your answers to the "Is This You?" questions tell a colorful story of metabolic dismay. Your lifestyle and eating habits have caused certain imbalances between very important hormones in your body, hormones that you must gain control of if you desire to lose fat and gain wellness and longevity. The 3+2 plan will enable you to regain healthy hormonal balance. The results you will experience while on this plan will be significant if not dramatic.

Now, let's talk about those hormonal imbalances. Based on the answers you gave, it seems that your body is having difficulty controlling the balance between insulin and glucagon. When you eat, your body usually produces too much insulin. When you do not eat, your body produces too much glucagon and cortisol. What this means to you is that when you do eat, you're likely to store some of the meal as fat, and if you don't eat, your body is going to use its muscle tissue as fuel—certainly both of these scenarios are unacceptable. These are common problems, however it will take a very uncommon approach to solve them.

The only way—and I mean the only way—to overcome these imbalances is with the right diet. There is no pill or potion to fix this. It is consistent beneficial food combinations that will wipe away these troubles and return your metabolism to "normal." The 3+2 will work for you in a number of ways:

- It will help to override the "starvation-protection mechanism" and turn on the calorie-burning switch in your body.
- It will keep insulin and glucagon in a near-perfect balance, by way of the specific 45/35/20 ratios, along with the frequent feedings and specific foods available.
- The 3+2 will lower cortisol levels by stabilizing the amount of glucose and amino acids in the bloodstream. Lower cortisol levels will allow greater fat loss and much more.

The 3+2 will be easy for you to follow and very easy to stick with for the long haul. By bringing balance back to your hormones, the 3+2 will remove cravings, increase energy, reduce fat, and improve the immune system and much more. Because you will feel so much better and look so much better while following the plan, it becomes very easy, in fact self-propelling. When you do not follow the plan, the difference in the way you feel will be obvious. It makes it easy—nearly effortless to get back on track.

I have designed the 3+2 for people just like you. This plan will get you out of the rut that you are now stuck in. This should be the easiest and most effective way of eating you have ever tried. Let's get started!

THE PLAN

The 3+2 Plan consists of three well-balanced meals that we will call breakfast, lunch, and dinner, and two additional smaller protein-based meals, which are consumed between breakfast and lunch and between lunch and dinner. The three daily meals will be very balanced meals that you could eat out with others. The two protein-based meals are only protein and can be eaten "on the go" or as a sit-down meal as well.

The three balanced meals you have each day should be spaced about 6 hours apart with the two protein-only meals in between. Each of the three balanced meals will need to contain the correct amounts of proteins, carbohydrates, and fats. The two protein-only meals will need to contain just the right amount of protein. Later in the chapter, you will see the formulas needed to calculate your portions for each meal and snack.

With this way of eating, you will never have to deny your hunger, never feel cravings for things you are "not allowed to have." The 45/35/20 ratio of carbohydrates, proteins, and fats together with the two 100% protein meals will bring the ideal balance between your metabolic hormones and create an environment favorable for energy, vitality, and fat reduction.

You will have a lengthy food list from which to choose the components of each meal. These are everyday foods and can be combined in hundreds of different ways, enabling you to eat at most any place you would like to. Yet these foods can also be combined very simply to create quick, easy meals at home. In fact, you will never have to cook a single meal unless you want to.

The 3+2 plan also allows many different free foods. These foods can be eaten as often as you like, with or without meals, and this allowance it makes this nutritional program very easy to adhere to. Particularly if you are a person who has a tendency to snack, this plan will allow you never to feel hungry, or feel that you are depriving yourself in any way. It is highly unlikely that you will not be able to stick with this plan because of cravings or a level of hunger that is out of control. After you have discovered what proportions make the ideal meal for you, there will be *a total absence of any food cravings*.

The 3+2 plan is very simple to follow, in that you are eating very normally and at times of the day when others around you are eating. The ratio of proteins, fats, and carbohydrates, the frequency of feeding, and especially those two protein snacks, will make that huge difference in the way you look and feel.

On the following pages you will find the formulas that must be used to figure out how much carbohydrates, proteins, and fats you will need to eat each meal. I have tried to keep this as simple as possible, so be patient and take your time. I recommend that you use the blanks like a workbook—yes, write in the book. It will be very easy to refer to this way. Once you have gone through the steps to determine what each meal will look like, you will be ready to get started.

YOUR BODY'S ENERGY (CALORIE) REQUIREMENTS

Basal Energy Requirement (BER)

The first step in designing your personal nutritional program is to determine your basal energy requirement (BER). The BER is the amount of energy (calories) your body requires in order to fuel its most basic functions. The BER is the approximate number of calories needed to breathe, think, pump blood through veins, etc.

There will be two different formulas for the BER. One for those who have had their body-fat measured, and one for those who have not. Once again, it is highly recommended that you have your body-fat measured prior to starting your nutritional plan. The BER is much more accurately determined if you know your fat percentage. If you have not had your fat measured, skip this section and proceed to the next.

The first step in determining the BER is to determine the amount of lean body weight you have. As we discussed in Chapter 1, lean body weight is the amount of your body that is not fat. It is the portion of your body that is composed of muscle, organs, bones, water, and other nonfat tissues.

For those who know their body-fat percentage, the formula to determine the amount of lean body weight is as follows. If you have not had your body-fat measured, skip this and go to the next section.

Body weight __*111*__ × Body-fat% __*17*__ = Fat Weight __*18.87*__

Body weight __*111*__ – Fat Weight __*18.87*__ = **Lean body weight (LBW)** __*92.13*__

Example

A person who weighs 100 lbs. with a body-fat of 15% will have 15 pounds of fat. This person would then have 85 lbs. of lean body weight (100 – 15 = 85). Once you have determined your lean body weight (LBW), the next step is to factor in your age.

Age Factor

Now take your lean body weight (LBW) and **multiply it by your age factor**. You will then have your basal energy requirement (BER).

- 50 years or older, the age factor is 13
- 40–50 years, the age factor is 14
- 20–40 years, the age factor is 15
- Up to 20 years, the age factor is 16

For example, a person with a LBW of 100 lbs., who is 36 years old, will have a BER of 1500. (100 × 15 = 1500)

Now, calculate your own BER.

LBW __*92*__ × Age factor __*14*__ = BER __*1290*__

Total Energy Requirement (TER)

Remember—the BER is the approximate number of calories your body will require to do nothing but exist. If you are active, you will need to adjust the BER to account for the energy expended during the activities. This number will be your total energy requirement or your TER. The total energy requirement (TER) is the approximate number of calories that your body will require to keep itself alive, *and* to perform the various activities of the day. In order to determine your TER, you will need to factor in your level of activity.

Activity Factor

The activity factor is used to approximate the number of calories you will need to consume to replace the amount of energy expended during exercise and other activities. Take your BER and add the appropriate number from the chart below. If you are not active, skip this calculation.

- If you participate in up to 30 minutes of exercise/activity per day, multiply your LBW by 2.
- If you participate in 30–60 minutes of exercise/activity per day, multiply your LBW by 3.
- If you participate in 60–90 minutes of exercise/activity per day, multiply your LBW by 4.

Example

A person who has a BER of 1500 calories and a lean body weight of 100 lbs., who exercises 60 minutes per day (activity factor = LBW multiplied by 3) will end up with a number of 1800. BER 1500 + Activity factor 300 = 1800. This number is the TER, or total energy requirement.

Now calculate your own activity factor.

LBW = __92__ × (2, 3, or 4) __3.5__ = Activity factor __322__

Now determine your total energy requirement (TER)

BER = _290_ + Activity factor _322_ = TER _1612_

(If you are inactive, your BER is the same as your TER.)

Adjusted Total Energy Requirement (ATER)

Remember—the TER is the approximate number of calories you would consume in a day if you wanted to maintain your current status. However, if you want to lose some body-fat, you will need to give your body a reason to use the fat as fuel. With few exceptions, this is accomplished by reducing the caloric intake to well below what your body requires to do the day's work. This adjusted calorie amount is known as the adjusted total energy requirement (ATER). As long as all the hormones are doing their jobs, and your metabolism is in a state of balance, the significant deficit of energy will cause your body to go into its fat reserves to get the missing energy. Hence, a reduction in body-fat.

To calculate your adjusted total energy requirement (ATER), simply take your TER and subtract 500.

Example

TER 1800 - 500 = 1300. (1300 is the ATER)

Now calculate your own adjusted total energy requirement (ATER).

TER _1612_ – 500 = _1112_ ATER

This number reflects the approximate number of calories you need to consume each day while attempting to reduce your level of body-fat. When you have lost all the fat you want to lose, use your TER as your daily caloric intake.

ENERGY (CALORIE) REQUIREMENTS WITHOUT A BODY-FAT MEASUREMENT

Caution: These formulas are only 70% accurate without a measurement of your body-fat percentage. *I recommend that you have your body-fat measured as soon as possible.*

Estimated Total Energy Requirement (ETER)

The estimated total energy requirement (ETER) is the approximate amount of energy (calories) that your body will need in a day to perform its basic functions (such as breathing and thinking), *in addition to* what it will require to complete the usual amount of exercise/activity.

Use the following guide to determine your ETER.

STEP ONE IS TO MULTIPLY YOUR BODY WEIGHT BY YOUR WEIGHT FACTOR.

Weight Factor

The weight factor is an approximation of the total amount of energy (calories) that a person of your weight, with an average amount of body-fat would need in a day just to maintain normal body function, such as breathing, thinking, etc. Use the following list to determine your weight factor.

- **Women** who weigh up to 120 lbs.—multiply your weight by *8.5*
- **Women** who weigh between 121 and 150 lbs.—multiply your weight by *8.25*
- **Women** who weigh between 151 and 200 lbs.—multiply your weight by *8*
- **Women** who weigh between 200 and 250 lbs.—multiply your weight by *7*
- **Women** who weigh more than 250 lbs.—multiply your weight by *6.5*
- **Men** who weigh up to 165 lbs.—multiply your weight by *10*
- **Men** who weigh 166 and 190 lbs.—multiply your weight by *9.5*
- **Men** who weigh more than 190 lbs.—multiply your weight by *9.25*

Now calculate your own weight factor.

Body weight __111__ × __8.5__ (weight factor) = __943.5__

STEP TWO IS TO APPLY YOUR ACTIVITY FACTOR.

Activity Factor

The activity factor is used to approximate the number of calories you will need to consume to replace the amount of energy expended during exercise and other activities. Take your weight factor and add the appropriate number from the chart below. If you are sedentary, skip this calculation.

- If you participate in up to 30 minutes of exercise/activity per day, add .5 calories per pound of body weight to your weight factor
- If you participate in 30–60 minutes of exercise/activity per day, add 1 calorie per pound of body weight to your weight factor
- If you participate in more than 60 minutes of exercise/activity per day, add 1.5 calories per pound of body weight to your weight factor

Example

A male who weighs 176 lbs. has a weight factor of 1672. (176 × 9.5 = 1672)

If he exercises 60 minutes per day, he has an activity factor of 176.(1 cal. × 176 lbs.=176)

So, his estimated total energy requirement ETER would be 1848. (1672 + 176 = 1848)

Now, calculate your own ETER.

Weight factor _____ + Activity factor _____ = ETER _____

YOUR IDEAL 3+2 MEAL

Now that you have determined the approximate number of calories you will need to consume each day, you'll need to divide that between the meals and snacks. You will also need to calculate how much carbohydrate, protein, and fat you'll need for each of the meals, along with the correct amount of protein for the protein only snacks.

Begin by taking your adjusted total energy requirement (ATER), or your estimated total energy requirement (ETER), and multiply it by 75% or .75. The number you come up with is the number of calories that will be divided between your three balanced meals.

ATER or ETER _____ × 75%(.75) = _____

Now, take that number and divide it by 3.

_____ ÷ 3 = _____ Calories per meal

(Each of the *three meals* will have this many calories.)

Now determine the approximate number of calories each of the *protein snacks* will contain.

ATER or ETER _____ × 25%(.25) = _____

Take that number and divide it by two.

_____ ÷ 2 = _____ Calories per protein snack

(This is the approximate number of calories each of the *protein snacks* will have.)

The next step is to determine the amount of protein, carbohydrate, and fat that each of the three meals will have. Take the number of calories each of the three meals will have, and multiply it by 45%, 35%, and 20%.

Calories per meal _____ × 45% = _____ Carbohydrate calories per meal

Now, because carbohydrate contains 4 calories per gram, divide the above number by 4 to determine the number of *grams* of carbohydrate per meal.

Carbohydrate calories per meal _____ ÷ 4 = _31_ **Grams of carbohydrate per meal**

Now you'll need to calculate the protein portion of each meal. Take the number of calories per meal and multiply it by 35%.

Calories per meal _____ × 35% = _____ Calories from protein for each meal

Because protein contains 4 calories per gram, divide the above number by 4 to determine the number of grams of protein per meal.

Protein calories per meal _____ ÷ 4 = _____ **Grams of protein per meal**

Now use the same formula to determine the fat content of each meal. Take the number of calories per meal and multiply it by 20%.

Calories per meal _____ × 20% = _____ Fat calories per meal

Now, because fat contains 9 calories per gram, take the number of fat calories per meal and divide it by 9—this will be the number of fat grams per meal.

Fat calories per meal _____ ÷ 9 = _____ **Grams of fat per meal**

Now let's calculate how much protein to have for the protein snacks.

Calories per protein snack _134_ ÷ 4 = _34_ **Grams of protein for each protein snack**

Now let's summarize the figures.

- **Grams of carbohydrate per meal** _____
- **Grams of protein per meal** _____
- **Grams of fat per meal** _____
- **Grams of protein for each protein snack** _____

PUTTING THE NUMBERS TO WORK

Now that you have successfully completed all the necessary calculations for the plan, its time to put them into action. Getting the right amounts of the different food groups is very important, so take your time and make sure you fully understand. You may need to read this part of the chapter two times, but once you really understand all these numbers, you will be equipped to have great success.

Portion Sizes

Determining your portion sizes is fairly easy, it just takes a couple of simple steps. Simply take the number of grams of carbohydrate, protein, or fat you need per meal, and divide it by the number of grams of carbohydrate per portion listed on the food list.

Example #1

Let's say that you need 21 grams of protein per meal. You have chosen to have turkey breast. Turkey breast contains 7 grams of protein per oz., so you would have 3 oz. (21 grams protein ÷ 7 grams protein/oz. = 3 oz.).

Example #2

If you needed 40 grams of carbohydrate per meal, and you chose to eat rice, you would have about one cup, because *cooked* rice contains about 37 grams carbohydrate per cup. (40 grams carbohydrate ÷ 37 grams carbohydrate in a cup = about one cup.)

All amounts listed on the food list are after cooking, except oatmeal, which is measured prior to cooking. I highly recommend that you weigh your portions a few times to become familiar with what amounts you should be eating. After just a few times weighing these foods, you will be able to "eyeball" the amounts.

If you do not see a particular food that you want to eat on the list, avoid the food for the first month. After that, simply determine how much carbohydrate, protein and fat the food contains, and calculate how much you need to have. Remember, though—avoid all non-listed foods for the first month.

Table 14.01

3+2 Plan Food List

PROTEINS

Chicken breast*
Turkey breast*
Venison*
Beefalo*
Buffalo*
Fish*
Shellfish*
Lamb
Veal
7% fat ground beef
Lean steaks
Lean cuts of pork
Canadian bacon
Ham
Average 7 grams protein/oz.

Egg whites*
3 grams protein each

Egg substitute*
Check label for protein content.

Nonfat cottage cheese *Average 3 grams protein/oz.*

Nonfat cheese
Average 9 grams protein/oz.

Tofu/Soy protein products
Check label for protein content. Watch for extra carbs and fats.

Protein powders*
*Microfiltered, ion-exchanged, predigested **whey** protein is best.*

CARBOHYDRATES

Yams/Sweet potatoes*
Red potatoes*
7 grams carbohydrate/oz.

Rice*
37 grams carbohydrate/cup

Oats*
27 grams carbohydrate 1/2 cup—uncooked

Beans/Lentils*
Average 35 grams carbohydrate/cup

Breads
Check label for carbohydrate content.

Bagels
Average 50 carbohydrates per bagel—check label.

Corn tortillas
Average 12 carbohydrates each

Flour tortillas
Average 20 carbohydrates each—check label.

Fruit
Average 35 carbohydrates per small piece

Melon
Average 45 carbohydrates per melon

Pasta
38 carbohydrates per cup

FATS

Safflower oil*
Sunflower oil*
Hemp oil*
Olive oil*
Canola oil*
Peanut oil*
Tahini oil*
Soybean oil*
Best not to cook oils 4 grams fat per tsp.

Nuts*
Check label for fat content.

Nut butters*
Average 3 grams fat per tsp.

Avocado*
3 grams fat per tbsp.

Olives*
1 gram fat each

Seeds*
Average 12 grams fat/oz.

Butter
*9 grams fat per pat
14 grams fat per tbsp.*

Mayonnaise
14 grams fat per tbsp.

Cream
5 grams fat per tbsp.

Cheese
Check label for fat content.

*Indicates best choices

All amounts listed are after cooking

Table 14.02

Free Foods List

The following foods are free foods. Unless otherwise noted, you can consume them at any time, with or without meals.

All vegetables *Except corn, peas, squash, carrots, beets*
Diet sodas *Avoid those containing phosphoric acid or caffeine or saccharin*
Diet flavored waters *Avoid those containing phosphoric acid or caffeine or saccharin*
Crystal Light
Regular coffee *Up to 2 cups per day*
Unlimited decaffeinated coffee *Preferably water processed*
Herbal teas *Caffeine-free*
Iced tea *Sugar-free; avoid saccharin; decaffeinated; green tea is best*
Swiss Miss diet cocoa *Up to 2 packets per day*
Sugar-free Jell-o
Sugar-free gum
Frozen yogurt *Maximum 4 oz., 2 times per week*
Gise Frozen Yogurt (800) 448-4473
Nonfat sour cream
Nonfat cream cheese
Nonfat mayonnaise
Nonfat salad dressing *Maximum of 2 tbsp. per day*
Citrus peels
Vinegars
Lemon and lime juice
Extracts
All dry seasonings and herbal seasonings
BBQ, Teriyaki, Mustard, Relish, Salsa, Ketchup, A-1,
Soy sauce (low sodium)

Note: Consumption of aspartame-containing food products is a personal decision. Much data exists to support its safety, but this continues to be a much-debated issue.

YOUR FIRST WEEK

It is an understatement to say that during your first week your body will be going through significant changes. You will be bringing back balance to what may have been unbalanced for most of your life. You may have never in your life arrived at what is correct for you. Because you are reading this book, you probably haven't. During this first week, you will be "kickstarting" your metabolism. As a result, you may be feeling certain things that are unusual for you. You may be depressed, or you may feel euphoric. You may get some acne, or you may eliminate the acne that you have. Your energy may soar, keeping you up at night, or you may feel totally lethargic for the first week. You will go through a number of metabolic changes that will result in symptoms that I am not able to predict. The only symptoms that should concern you are those that involve pain, disorientation or discomfort. Consult your physician immediately if you have any concern.

What you must do is keep moving forward, no matter what. No matter how you feel. I liken this to the way you would drive a car. You place your foot on the gas pedal, and the car begins to move forward. If you hold the gas pedal down, the car travels faster and faster. As the car travels faster, it also uses up more fuel. This fuel consumption allows the car to travel even faster. What happens when you let your foot off the gas pedal? The car slows back down. In other words, if you deprive yourself of food, you will not have enough gas fueling your engine. If, because you feel like you are eating too much, or eating foods that don't make sense, you change your plan in any way, *you will never get over the hump*. You will never reach freeway speeds, and you will be stuck on side-streets forever. So keep going forward no matter what. For this first week you will have to go on faith. Don't let up, and you will be well on your journey.

HELPFUL HINTS

You must not miss meals. If you do not eat **three** times a day and have your protein shakes at least 80% of the time, you will not succeed.

If you happen to overeat one meal, do **not** *undereat during the next meal*. In other words, do not alter any meal, based on a mistake you made on the meal prior to that, or in anticipation of a meal that is ahead of you. By doing this you will have ruined two meals. Each meal is its own separate entity, and is not reliant on any other meal. Each meal is like taking a medicine that we are trying to get an effect from, that will wear off in a few hours, so we would take that medicine again. If you change the medicine once, would you change the medicine again to account for that? No. You can't double up, you can't cut it in half. You will simply be ruining a half of your day instead of a quarter of your day. Even in cases of extreme over-eating, the next meal is exactly as it should be. We are attempting to create an environment for your metabolism. Allow that environment to be as stable as possible. The same applies to undereating. Do not eat more the next time.

You've heard it a hundred times, but I'll say it again. You must drink enough water. If you are dehydrated, you will not burn fat. End of story. Water is necessary in the process of not only fat reduction, but every metabolic process. If you are not drinking enough water, you will fail. You should be urinating about ten times per day for your fat to remove itself from your body. If you are not in the bathroom more than you think you should be, you are not in there enough. Drink at least eight 12-oz. glasses of water each day.

Another suggestion I would make would be to purchase a food scale. Don't assume that you know anything. Even if you have been on a program where you had to weigh your food. It is vital that you are getting the proper amount of food in the correct ratios for this to work for you. You don't want to be, and you don't need to be measuring everything that you eat. However, for the first week or so, I want you to get a better idea of what your portion size will look like. If you have determined, by using "The Perfect Portion," that you need 6 oz. of protein with each meal, weigh that out before and after cooking. Put it in your bowl of salad or on the plate, so that you can be accustomed to what that portion size looks like. Give yourself that edge, you'll thank me for it down the road. If you are unable to locate a scale, call toll-free (888) 663–2881.

For this or any other plan, preparation is key. Know that if you will be in the middle of nowhere when mealtime rolls around, that you will have brought something to eat with you. If you know that you will be in the middle of a meeting when mealtime comes around, bring a meal replacement in with you, so that you do not activate your starvation-protection mechanism. You don't have to eat a meal, you just have to ingest the proper amounts of carbohydrate, protein, and fat. Prepare a thermos full of a meal replacement drink, to have throughout the day. Don't go out into the world everyday, and just expect that the right food will be there. It won't be there. Think ahead. Plan for your success.

Make sure you are getting enough protein. Most menu items will not have the necessary protein content. You must learn to order additional portions, or let them know exactly how much you need. You must make an Olympian effort to get enough protein.

Foods must be eaten together at the same time to bring about the desired results. A major point of eating in this prescribed manner is to stimulate or repress the production of specific hormones that make up the metabolism. To foster this hormone activity, these foods must be ingested as a whole. Do not, under any circumstances, have a protein without the fat portion of the meal or vice versa. These food groups will always be consumed at the same time, or eating will have the exact opposite outcome than the results you desire.

It is most beneficial to have vegetables with each meal. Vegetables will not only eliminate any trace of carbohydrate craving, but will also be very filling, and regulate the bowels very successfully. In addition to these benefits, many vegetables are high in the EFAs and contain special nutrients that are tremendously beneficial to the human body.

Do not have more than two alcoholic beverages per week. If you have a couple (two) glasses of alcohol per week, it should have no effect. Your body will absorb it, and you won't even see it. Any greater alcohol consumption and it is a ball and chain wrapped around your waist that you are dragging with you 24 hours a day. The alcoholic portion of any beverage you consume *will* be converted to body-fat. For women this body-fat is gathered at the back of the arms, the hips, and just below the belly button. For men, it seems to gather between the chest and the pelvic area.

The correct supplementation program can dramatically enhance your results. My experience with thousands of clients has proven that the proper diet combined with a well-designed supplementation program will provide an average of approximately *30% increased rate of fat reduction*. In addition to faster and greater fat reduction, you can achieve a stronger immune system, higher energy levels, and most importantly a higher success rate of maintenance. You will find a comprehensive guide to these supplements in Chapter 5.

Meal replacement "Protein bars" are an excellent way to have a meal in a hurry or on-the-go. Depending on which plan you have chosen, you will be required to eat 4–7 times per day. In many cases, this is a difficult task, one that can be made much easier with the option of having a meal replacement bar. Just open the wrapper and eat your meal—it is as easy as that. You can use these bars as often as needed, as long as they contain the appropriate amounts of proteins, carbohydrates, and fats. There are many of these bars available. The trick is to find the bar that contains the necessary amounts of proteins, carbohydrates, and fats for your plan. To find the right bar, just go to your local health food store and either look at the labels yourself, or ask for help. You can also call (888) 663-2881 to have some of the right bars sent to you.

That's it! Good luck! Go get started now.

## 15

THE INSULIN BUSTER

EASE

*T*his is a very simple and easy to follow diet. In this diet, there is no formal structure. You do not have to weigh or measure foods. There is simply a list of foods that you can eat while you are on the program. On this list, you can have all the food you want, whenever you want, in any quantity. It couldn't be easier.

EATING OUT

This is an ideal plan if you eat out often. The foods that are acceptable on this diet are typically the foods that you would believe are making America fat, but we will use them to make us thin.

RATE OF FAT LOSS

One can expect to lose between two and six pounds of body-fat per week. Most will lose between three and four pounds of body-fat a week.

ENERGY LEVEL

Your energy level will be steady from the moment you wake up until you go to bed, without experiencing slumps in the mid-afternoon.

DURATION

The recommended duration of the insulin buster is 4 weeks. This will be just enough of a primer for your body to be ready to go on to another plan. This plan is intended only as a short-term "shock" to the metabolism. After the 4-week period, re-read the "Is This You?" questions and determine what plan you will follow next.

YOUR UNIQUE METABOLISM

Welcome to Hormones 101. In this class you will be learning about hormones, including insulin, glucagon, cortisol, human growth hormone (HGH), and others, which are at the root of many of your troubles.

Your answers to the "Is This You?" questions paint a picture of *significant* problems with the management of insulin, glucagon, and cortisol within your body. It seems that your body is now, and has been for quite some time, producing more than normal amounts of insulin, too little glucagon, and far too much cortisol. This *significant* hormonal pandemonium has caused widespread dysfunction in your body.

Among your problems, the poor control of insulin is really the major player. This type of significant insulin management problem is a common problem and has even been labeled by the medical community. They call it Syndrome X. Many insurance companies recognize this level of dysinsulinism as a treatable illness. Check with your doctor.

If you have read Chapter 2, you already know of insulin's awesome power and relative danger. For those of you who did not read Chapter 2, I recommend that you do so at this time. For now, we will go ahead and go over the basics of insulin.

Insulin is a hormone secreted by the pancreas. It is an essential hormone, in that you cannot survive without it. Insulin helps your body regulate the amount of glucose (blood sugar) in the bloodstream. Insulin transports the glucose into cells where it can be used for energy and repair of the cell. If your cells do not need all the glucose that insulin brings to them, the extra will be stored away as fat. Insulin also transports proteins and fats, but this is not as important for our discussion today.

Your answers suggest that when you eat normal meals or foods, your body responds by producing far too much insulin. The extra insulin will take even a small amount of glucose and store it away as fat. This faulty insulin reaction necessitates your complete avoidance of carbohydrates and sugars. This is due to the fact that these types of foods are the most likely to cause your body to produce the extra insulin.

Oversecretion of insulin can cause a wide array of illnesses, including diabetes, obesity, cardiovascular disease, problems with eyesight, high blood pressure, and many others.

I have designed the insulin buster specifically to help people overcome significant insulin management problems. The insulin buster is not a long-term plan. It usually takes 45 days or less to regain control of insulin levels within the body. The insulin buster is a short-term, aggressive approach to eliminating insulin management problems.

The insulin buster works in a number of ways:

1. It effectively eliminates most insulin from the blood, allowing your body time to recover from the effects of high insulin.
2. It keeps blood glucose levels very low, which promotes the formation of ketones. Ketones promote fat burning.
3. By bringing balance to hormones, the insulin buster will eliminate all food cravings, making it easy to stick with the plan.
4. The insulin buster also teaches your body to use fat as fuel and not always glucose.
5. The presence of ketones keeps energy levels high, hormones balanced, and your fat-burning switch turned on full.

The insulin buster will prove to be very useful to you in your quest for leanness and wellness. It is, in my opinion, the best way for a person who has this level of insulin problems to begin to eliminate them.

THE PLAN

The insulin buster is a short-term plan. I recommend that you follow it for only 4 weeks. The insulin buster is a high-fat diet. Most of the calories that you will ingest on this program, typically between 50% and 70% of the total amount of the food you will eat, will be comprised of fat.

You are probably thinking, "Wait a minute. How do I get thin from eating fat?" You have probably learned in the past that fat makes you fat. Nothing could be further from the truth. Fat does not, nor does it have the potential to, make you fat. Insulin makes you fat. Fat does not promote any significant production of insulin, carbohydrates do. Carbohydrates have much more potential to create body fat than fat does. Surprisingly, this particular diet also has benefited a large majority of individuals who suffer from high blood pressure, diabetes, and high cholesterol levels. The food combination of this diet focuses on protein and fat. When you consume fat and protein together there is very little insulin production. Therefore, fat cannot be converted into body-fat and instead it is used to fuel muscle and organ tissue. For example, a donut or a Snickers bar, which are made up of carbohydrates *and* fat, stimulate the production of insulin, and that insulin secretion stores the carbohydrates *and* the fat into your body-fat. As an example, one could eat 1000 calories of pure fat and put very little of it away as body-fat. Conversely, eating 1000 calories of donuts would result in large amounts of fat storage.

On this plan, calories are not the issue. The right food at the right time is the issue. On this particular diet, anytime is the right time. The right time is when your body tells you that you are hungry. When we eat, we are basically fueling a motor, and on this plan we will be burning fuel at a very high rate. Like your car, when your motor runs out of fuel, it stops. If you were driving down the highway and your gas gauge was on E, you wouldn't just keep driving . . . you would pull over and get some gas. Why would it be any different with your body? If your body tells you that it needs energy, and you fail to provide it with fuel, the motor will shut down.

You cannot break rule #1 on this diet:

YOU MUST EAT WHEN YOU ARE HUNGRY. If you get hungry at 2:30 in the afternoon, you must be eating by 2:45 or sooner. Let your level of hunger determine how much food you should have on this plan. If you grossly overeat on this program, you may not get great results, but you will not become any fatter.

This nutritional program is based on the eating habits of hunter tribes, whose diets were comprised mostly of meat, and as a result are very lean. This plan was actually discovered in the early 1900s. When it became a formalized "diet," it was structured and produced for epileptics and other people who were suffering from seizure activity. After watching patients get better, doctors also noticed that their patients were getting leaner. At that time, these doctors did not know about insulin, or have the benefit of what science has taught us in the last century. We now know that by being on a high-fat diet, the body can be driven into a state called ketosis. By producing substances called ketones, which travel through the bloodstream and up to the brain to effect the centers where seizures originate, the patients of the early 1900s showed a marked improvement in their condition.

Ketosis was also the condition that enabled these patients to decrease their body fat. Simply put, ketones are partially burned fat cells. As we discussed in Chapter 2, a fat cell is made up of three fatty acid molecules and a glycerin molecule. When you are in a state of ketosis, the body breaks apart the fat cell, and may only use one or two of those molecules for energy. The remainder or the waste of that cell is called a ketone. Ketones can supply energy to all systems of the body. In this light, ketones are an excellent source of energy, and act almost the same way as sugar does, but do not raise insulin levels like sugars do. What this means to you is that your energy can stay high without eating any carbohydrates.

Ketogenic diets have received much bad press. This is due to the fact that ketosis is a dangerous condition for diabetics, and most of what is known about ketosis comes from this arena. For healthy people, ketosis is a great way to raise glucagon and lower insulin levels. Ketosis is an excellent short-term approach to losing fat and maintaining muscle, while reversing some of your insulin management problem.

On this plan, you will also find that your body won't crave sugar. By burning stored body-fat to produce ketones, you will trick the body into believing that you are eating plenty of sugar. You will also find that you will lose fat very rapidly on this plan.

On this nutritional program, you should measure your ketone level, so that you can insure that you have achieved a state of ketosis. You will measure your ketone level *twice per day* (once in the morning, once in the evening) with a product that is readily available, and can be found in your local pharmacy. This product is called a ketone measuring stick (Ketostix). Ketone measuring sticks are paper strips with a cloth reagent attached to the end. When the cloth is dipped into your urine, it will turn a certain color. That color will correspond with a chart on the back of the bottle, and will tell you your ketone level. You want to be between "trace" (light pink) and "moderate" (light purple) all of the time.

If you are *not* in trace and are in the negative, or if you are over moderate and into *heavy* ketosis, you have gone into an area that is not desirable and you will need to modify your program. If your stick shows "negative," you are most probably eating carbohydrates that you are not aware of. Some additive, spice, or food you are eating is sweetened with sugar and/or caffeine is interfering with the process of ketosis. This means that carbohydrates are being burned for energy and you are not burning fat. So take a really close look at your food before you decide that this isn't working for you. You can raise your ketone levels by exercising.

If, after searching your diet high and low for hidden sugars and carbohydrates, you still come up with no ketones and no reason for it, you should stop and revisit the "Is This You?" questions and begin an alternate plan. This is because a small portion of the population will have an extremely difficult time achieving a state of ketosis. These people need more guidance than I can give within a chapter.

If your stick reads purple, or heavy, meaning that you have a very high level of ketone production, either you are not eating enough or you are eating *way too much* fat. Chances are that you are *not eating enough* fat, and as a result, you are burning off muscle. Having such a large amount of ketones in the blood is not desirable, so figure it out and bring your ketones into the trace to moderate range ASAP.

Most ketone measuring products will have a chart that looks similar to this. Shades are pink to purple.

Chart 15.01

Keytone Chart

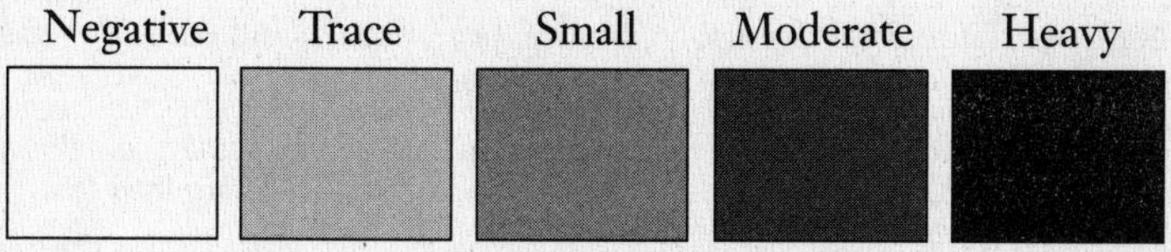

Negative	Trace	Small	Moderate	Heavy

Table 15.01

The Insulin Buster Food List

What follows is a list of foods that you can eat while you are on this program.

MEATS

Beef, pork, lamb, veal*, venison*, moose, bear, ostrich and emu. *Any meat is acceptable, even products like bacon and salami!*

> **Please Note:** Be careful about choosing cured meats that contain sodium nitrate and sodium nitrite. It has recently been determined that these ingredients are carcinogens.

POULTRY

Chicken* and turkey* with or without the skin.

FISH

Salmon*, halibut*, mackerel*, lobster*, clams, scallops*, swordfish*, tuna*, shrimp*—*Again, any fish, shellfish, or crustacean, in any combination.*

FOWL

Quail, duck, pheasant, and goose. *If I left any out, please feel free to eat them.*

CHEESE

Bleu, swiss*, cheddar, jack, havarti, brie, feta*, goat cheese*, camembert, roquefort, munster, mozzarella*, farmers, and string. *Put the entire state of Wisconsin in your fridge, any cheese will do.*

PROTEIN DRINKS

Ion-exchanged, predigested, microfiltered whey protein. Egg white protein would by the next best choice.

FATS

Butter, cream, mayonnaise, fatty broths and stocks, oils of any kind (olive, safflower, sunflower, and flax oils are preferred), pure whipped cream, olives, and limit yourself to only ½ avocado per day. *(Note: Fry oils as seldom as possible.)*

VEGGIES

You may have a maximum of 3 cups of these vegetables each day.
Celery, radiccio, chives, jicama, parsley, cucumber, radishes, sprouts, peppers, mushrooms, hearts of palm, onions, scallions, spinach, asparagus, string beans, cabbage, cauliflower and eggplant.

You may not have caffeine.

(* indicates best choice)

Table 15.02

Free Foods for the Insulin Buster

Vinegar	Diet beverages
Lemon juice	Decaffeinated coffee
Lime juice	Sparkling water
Mustard	Water
Garlic	Iced tea
Mushrooms	Herbal tea
Onions	Dry seasonings (Herbal, etc.)
Scallions	Salt
Cucumber	Pepper
Lettuce	Sugar-free Jell-o
Citrus peels	Sugar-free gum
Chili peppers	

THE RULES

1. **Eat when you are hungry.**
2. **Refer to rule #1.**
3. **Eat as many meals as you desire.**
4. **Do not overeat. Eat only until you are satisfied.**
5. **Refer to rule #1.**
6. **Drink plenty of fluids. A good place to start would be a gallon of water per day.**
7. **You are not on a low-fat diet—eat fat!**
8. **No carbohydrates!**
9. **One time per week, you should have a carbohydrate-containing food. This is not a cheat, but a stimulus to your metabolism and will help your body continue to benefit from the plan.**
10. **You must measure your ketones twice per day and maintain trace to moderate ketosis.**
11. **You must not have any caffeinated beverages. Keep your caffeine intake as low as possible (you won't miss it).**
12. **30 minutes of cardiovascular exercise per day, four days per week will add 40% to your result.**

This plan is very simple. You may not have carbohydrates, but you may have as much of the other foods as you like. After a short time, you will lose your craving for carbohydrates. There are no restricted amounts on the foods you may eat, so let your hunger and ketone levels decide your portions. Let your body decide if you need 2 ounces or 16 ounces. You can't go wrong. Please drink plenty of liquids, and avoid caffeine like the plague.

YOUR FIRST WEEK

It is an understatement to say that during your first week, your body will be going through significant changes. You will be bringing back balance to what may have been unbalanced for your entire life. You may have never in your life arrived at what is correct for you. Because you are reading this book, you probably haven't. During this first week, you will be rearranging the metabolism. As a result, you may be feeling certain things that are unusual for you. You may be depressed, or you may feel euphoric. You may get some acne, or you may eliminate the acne that you have. Your energy may soar, keeping you up at night, or you may feel totally lethargic for the first week. You will go through a number of metabolic changes that will result in symptoms that I am not able to predict.

What you must do is keep moving forward, no matter what. No matter how you feel. I liken this to the way you would drive a car. You place your foot on the gas pedal, and the car begins to move forward. If you hold the gas pedal down, the car travels faster and faster. As the car travels faster, it also uses up more fuel. This fuel consumption allows the car to travel even faster. What happens when you let your foot off the gas pedal? The car slows back down. In other words, if you deprive yourself of food, you will not have enough gas in your engine. If you feel like you are eating too much, or change the way you should be eating because you are feeling a certain way, *you will* **never** *get over the hump*. You will never reach freeway speeds, and you will be stuck on side-streets forever. So keep going forward no matter what. For this first week you will have to go on faith. Don't let up, and you will be well on your journey.

HELPFUL HINTS

Make sure that you stay between "trace" and "moderate" on the ketone-measuring sticks. If you are out of this range, you will not be successful on this plan. When your ketones show negative, you must search for hidden carbohydrates or sugars, or eat less. When your ketones show too high, you must eat more.

You've heard it a hundred times, but I'll say it again. You must drink enough water. If you are dehydrated, you will not burn fat. End of story. Water is necessary in the process of not only fat reduction, but every metabolic process. If you are not drinking enough water, you will fail. You should be urinating about ten times per day for your fat to remove itself from your body. If you are not in the bathroom more than you think you should be, you are not in there enough. Drink at least eight 12-oz. glasses of water each day.

For this or any other plan, preparation is key. Know that if you will be in the middle of nowhere when mealtime rolls around, that you will have brought something to eat with you. If you know that you will be in the middle of a meeting when mealtime comes around, bring a meal replacement in with you, so that you do not activate your starvation protection mechanism. Prepare a thermos full of protein drink, to have throughout the day. Don't go out into the world everyday and just expect that the right food will be there. It won't be there. Think ahead. Plan for your success.

Do not have more than two alcoholic beverages per week. If you have a couple (two) glasses of alcohol per week, it should have no effect. Your body will absorb it, and you won't even see it. Any greater alcohol consumption and it is a ball and chain wrapped around your waist that you are dragging with you 24 hours a day. The alcoholic portion of any beverage you consume *will* be converted to body-fat. For women this body-fat is gathered at the back of the arms, the hips, and just below the belly button. For men, it seems to gather between the chest and the pelvic area.

If you are craving carbohydrates, you have not eaten enough protein and fat. When you are consuming enough protein and fat, you will not have any cravings. Having any cravings for any carbohydrate food is merely a signal from your body that you are definitely undereating.

The correct supplementation program can dramatically enhance your results. My experience with thousands of clients has proven that the proper diet combined with a well-designed supplementation program, will provide an average of approximately 30% increased rate of fat reduction. In addition to faster and greater fat reduction, you can achieve a stronger immune system, higher energy levels, and most importantly a higher success rate of maintenance. You will find a comprehensive guide to these supplements in Chapter 5.

Meal replacement "Protein bars" are an excellent way to have a meal in a hurry or on-the-go. Depending on which plan you have chosen, you will be required to eat 4–7 times per day. In many cases, this is a difficult task, one that can be made much easier with the option of having a meal replacement bar. Just open the wrapper and eat your meal—it is as easy as that. You can use these bars as often as needed, as long as they contain the appropriate amounts of proteins, carbohydrates, and fats. There are many of these bars available. The trick is to find the bar that contains the necessary amounts of proteins, carbohydrates, and fats for your plan. To find the right bar, just go to your local health food store and either look at the labels yourself, or ask for help. You can also call (888) 663-2881 to have some of the right bars sent to you.

Within two weeks you will feel outstanding!

## 16

THE 40/40/20 PLAN

EASE

*T*his nutritional program is one of the easiest and most accommodating plans you could possibly be on. The food choices on this plan are simple with easy to find foods that are available almost everywhere.

EATING OUT

Eating out is very easy. The foods that you will be eating while you are on this plan are readily available, and you will find them on virtually every menu in virtually every restaurant. The only difficulty you may encounter is that, at times, you will have to order an extra protein portion to meet your required needs.

RATE OF FAT LOSS

For those who use the proper portions, the rate of fat loss, relative to anything that you have ever done before will be phenomenal. You should and will experience anywhere from 1 to 4 pounds of body-fat reduction per week.

ENERGY

Your energy will be incredible, and will be sustained throughout the day. You will experience this energy level from the moment you wake up, and feel that same level of energy consistently throughout the day, until just before bedtime.

DURATION

You are the person for this diet. This is not a temporary solution, but rather, a permanent adjustment for the manner in which you should eat for the rest of your life. After you have eliminated unwanted body-fat, the only adjustment you would make would be the total number of calories you need on a daily basis.

YOUR UNIQUE METABOLISM

The situation could definitely be much worse. Your answers to the "Is This You?" questions suggest that you are in the early stages of metabolic disaster. Your body is fighting a battle that it is losing, but it is still putting up a good fight. If you do not change your ways in a hurry, and these problems inside your body continue, you will lose that war. The problems I am referring to are the imbalances between the hormones that make up your metabolism. When you eat, your body does not respond with a normal productive secretion of metabolic hormones. Insulin is slightly elevated, glucagon is slightly depressed, cortisol is going up, and HGH is going down. Your cells are not responding to various stimuli as well as they should be. Your body is quick to store fat and hesitant to burn any. Again, these problems are in the beginning stages and you will not need to be on an aggressive plan to bring back normal function, but if you fail to correct these problems now, you will pay the price later. You have found this book at the right time.

The 40/40/20 will effect positive changes in your metabolism in many ways:

1. Consistent intake of a 40/40/20 ratio will provide a stable blood sugar level, eliminating sugar cravings and increasing energy levels.
2. The 40/40/20 ratio will help to lower insulin, raise glucagon and HGH, and eliminate much of the excess cortisol from your blood.
3. The high quality proteins, carbohydrates, and fats will bring countless benefits to your body.
4. The consistent balance of the 40/40/20 will re-teach your body how to effectively process the foods you eat.
5. The 40/40/20 ratio will educate your cells on how to utilize body-fat as the primary fuel source.

It will be relatively easy for you to bring balance back to your metabolism. It will require very simple changes to the way you combine normal foods. The 40/40/20 combination will cause a shift in the way your body processes the foods you eat. Right now, 40/40/20 is the key to your metabolic turnaround.

Chances are that you will be able to continue this plan long term. This plan will not only *get you lean*, but will also *keep you that way*. The 40/40/20 works.

Now let's get started.

THE PLAN

The 40/40/20 plan requires that you eat four meals per day, which are spaced apart by about four hours. You should have breakfast, lunch, a mid-afternoon meal, and dinner. The food choices on this plan are widely available and popular foods that you will be able to find almost anywhere. The meals that you eat will be made up of 40% carbohydrate, 40% protein, and 20% fat. There is also a lengthy list of foods that are "free" foods. In between, during, and in addition to the four meals you must eat per day, you may draw on this list of "free" foods any time you desire. You may have these foods as often as you like, at any time you like.

The prescribed ratio of 40% carbohydrate, 40% protein, and 20% fat is truly a balanced meal. Your diet is designed in this way because your particular metabolism requires the high energy afforded by eating a larger percentage of carbohydrates, and an equally high intake of protein in relation to fat. This plan allows you a lot of freedom, in that, there are a wide range of food choices that will not preclude you from eating out of a box, or having to shop at a specialty health food store for groceries.

What you will accomplish in eating balanced meals at regular intervals will be to achieve a significantly higher energy level that will stay at that level, and last throughout the day until just before bedtime. You will also see improvements in your skin and hair quality. Your thought process will be much clearer. Creativity will return. The fogginess that is undoubtedly in your head now will leave, and a crisp and clear thought process will replace it. Short-term and long-term memory will vastly improve. Your bowel movements will improve. The frequency of urination for most people will go up to about ten times per day. This is a very good thing, as you will be voiding unwanted body-fat byproducts in the process.

By eating a balanced meal at regular intervals, you will be effectively balancing all the hormones that are at work when you eat. The most significant change will be the additional protein you will be eating. For you the perfect meal may be an entirely new concept that may include some new foods. You will be processing these new food choices in a very efficient manner. You will become a walking meal clock, in that, hunger will be present only just before mealtime. You will wake up hungry in the morning, and you should eat breakfast before you leave the house. (Unless, of course, you are leaving the house to eat breakfast.) This will eliminate your need for the instant energy gratification that sweets have afforded you in the past. You will not even have to think about what time it is. After two or three days, you will know what time it is by your level of hunger.

The first step in designing your own 40/40/20 plan is to determine the correct number of calories to consume each meal, and how to break those calories up into the prescribed 40/40/20 ratio.

Use the following formulas to determine your individual caloric requirements.

YOUR BODY'S ENERGY (CALORIE) REQUIREMENTS

Basal Energy Requirement (BER)

The first step in designing your personal nutritional program is to determine your basal energy requirement (BER). The BER is the amount of energy your body requires in order to fuel its most basic functions. The BER is the approximate number of calories needed to breathe, think, pump blood through veins, etc.

There will be two different formulas for the BER. One for those who have had their body-fat measured, and one for those who have not. Once again, it is highly recommended that you have your body-fat measured prior to starting your nutritional plan.

The BER is much more accurately determined if you know your fat percentage. If you have not had your fat measured, skip this section and proceed to the next.

The first step in determining the BER is to determine the amount of lean body weight you have. As we discussed in Chapter 1, lean body weight is the amount of your body that is not fat. It is the portion of your body that is composed of muscle, organs, bones, water, and other nonfat tissues.

For those who know their body-fat percentage, the formula to determine the amount of lean body weight is as follows. If you have not had your body-fat measured, skip this and go to the next section.

Body weight __115__ × Body-fat% __19.5__ = Fat weight __22.4__

Body weight _____ – Fat weight _____ = **Lean body weight (LBW)** __92.6__

Example

A person who weighs 100 lbs. with a body-fat of 15% will have 15 pounds of fat. This person would then have 85 lbs. Of lean body weight (100 − 15 = 85).

Once you have determined your lean body weight (LBW), the next step is to factor in your age.

Age Factor

Now take your lean body weight (LBW) and **multiply it by your age factor**. You will then have your basal energy requirement (BER).

- 50 years or older, the age factor is 13
- 40–50 years, the age factor is 14
- 20–40 years, the age factor is 15
- Up to 20 years, the age factor is 16

For example, a person with a LBW of 100 lbs., who is 36 years old, will have a BER of 1500 (100 × 15 = 1500).

Now, calculate your own BER.

LBW _92.6_ × Age factor _14_ = BER _1296_

Total Energy Requirement (TER)

Remember—the BER is the approximate number of calories your body will require to do nothing but exist. If you are active, you will need to adjust the BER to account for the energy expended during the activities. This number will be your total energy requirement or your TER. The total energy requirement (TER) is the approximate number of calories that your body will require to keep itself alive, *and* to perform the various activities of the day. In order to determine your TER, you will need to factor in your level of activity.

Activity Factor

The activity factor is used to approximate the number of calories you will need to consume to replace the amount of energy expended during exercise and other activities. Take your BER and add the appropriate number from the list below. If you are not active, skip this calculation.

- If you participate in up to 30 minutes of exercise/activity per day, multiply your LBW by 2.
- If you participate in 30–60 minutes of exercise/activity per day, multiply your LBW by 3.
- If you participate in 60–90 minutes of exercise/activity per day, multiply your LBW by 4.

Example

A person who has a BER of 1500 calories and a lean body weight of 100 lbs., who exercises 60 minutes per day (activity factor = LBW multiplied by 3) will end up with a number of 1800. BER 1500 + Activity factor 300 = 1800. This number is the TER, or total energy requirement.

Now calculate your own activity factor.

LBW = __92.6__ × (2, 3, or 4) _____ = Activity factor __231__

Now determine your total energy requirement (TER).

BER = __1296__ + Activity factor _____ = TER __1527__

If you are inactive, your BER is the same as your TER.

Adjusted Total Energy Requirement (ATER)

Remember—the TER is the approximate number of calories you would consume in a day if you wanted to maintain your current status. However, if you want to lose some body-fat, you will need to give your body a reason to use the fat as fuel. With few exceptions, this is accomplished by reducing the caloric intake to well below what your body requires to do the day's work. This adjusted calorie amount is known as the adjusted total energy requirement (ATER). As long as all the hormones are doing their jobs, and your metabolism is in a state of balance, the significant deficit of energy will cause your body to go into its fat reserves to get the missing energy. Hence, a reduction in body-fat.

To calculate your adjusted total energy requirement (ATER), simply take your TER and subtract 500.

Example

TER 1800 - 500 = 1300. (1300 is the ATER)

Now calculate your own adjusted total energy requirement (ATER).

TER _____ – 500 = _1027_ ATER

This number reflects the approximate number of calories you need to consume each day while attempting to reduce your level of body-fat.

ENERGY (CALORIE) REQUIREMENTS WITHOUT A BODY-FAT MEASUREMENT

Caution: These formulas are only 70% accurate without a measurement of your body-fat percentage. *I recommend that you have your body-fat measured as soon as possible.*

Estimated Total Energy Requirement (ETER)

The estimated total energy requirement (ETER) is the approximate amount of energy (calories) that your body will need in a day to perform its basic functions (such as breathing and thinking), *in addition to* what it will require to complete the usual amount of exercise/activity.

Use the following guide to determine your ETER.

STEP ONE IS TO MULTIPLY YOUR BODY WEIGHT BY YOUR WEIGHT FACTOR.

Weight Factor

The weight factor is an approximation of the total amount of energy (calories) that a person of your weight, with an average amount of body-fat would need in a day just to maintain normal body function, such as breathing, thinking, etc. Use the following list to determine your weight factor.

- **Women** who weigh up to 120 lbs.—multiply your weight by *8.5*
- **Women** who weigh between 121 and 150 lbs.—multiply your weight by *8.25*
- **Women** who weigh between 151 and 200 lbs.—multiply your weight by *8*
- **Women** who weigh between 200 and 250 lbs.—multiply your weight by *7*
- **Women** who weigh more than 250 lbs.—multiply your weight by *6.5*
- **Men** who weigh up to 165 lbs.—multiply your weight by *10*
- **Men** who weigh 166 and 190 lbs.—multiply your weight by *9.5*
- **Men** who weigh more than 190 lbs.—multiply your weight by *9.25*

Now calculate your own weight factor.

Body weight _____ × _____ (weight factor) = _____

STEP TWO IS TO APPLY YOUR ACTIVITY FACTOR.

Activity Factor

The activity factor is used to approximate the number of calories you will need to consume to replace the amount of energy expended during exercise and other activities. Take your weight factor and add the appropriate number from the list below. If you are sedentary, skip this calculation.

- If you participate in up to 30 minutes of exercise/activity per day, add .5 calories per pound of body weight to your weight factor.
- If you participate in 30–60 minutes of exercise/activity per day, add 1 calorie per pound of body weight to your weight factor.
- If you participate in more than 60 minutes of exercise/activity per day, add 1.5 calories per pound of body weight to your weight factor.

Example

A male who weighs 176 lbs. has a weight factor of 1672 (176 × 9.5 = 1672). If he exercises 60 minutes per day, he has an activity factor of 176 (1 cal × 176 lbs.=176). So, his estimated total energy requirement ETER would be 1848 (1672 + 176 = 1848).

Now, calculate your own ETER.

Weight factor _977_ + Activity factor _15_ = ETER _1092_

This is the approximate number of calories you will consume each day.

1113

YOUR IDEAL 40/40/20 MEAL

Remember—the ETER is the approximate number of calories to be consumed each day, but you will need to divide those calories between the four meals.

Begin by taking your adjusted total energy requirement (ATER) or your estimated total energy requirement (ETER) and dividing it by 4. This number will be calories per meal.

Adjusted

ATER or ETER _1027_ ÷ 4 = _256_ **Calories per meal**

1113   *248*

Now that you have determined the approximate number of calories to consume each meal, you'll have to break that down to grams of carbohydrate, protein, and fat per meal.

Take the number of calories each of the three meals will have, and multiply it by 40%, 40%, and 20%.

Calories per meal _256_ × 40% = _102_ Carbohydrate calories per meal

Now, because carbohydrate contains 4 calories per gram, divide the above number by 4 to determine the number of *grams* of carbohydrate per meal.

Carbohydrate calories per meal _192_ ÷ 4 = _25.6_ **Grams of carbohydrate per meal**

Now you'll need to calculate the protein portion of each meal. Take the number of calories per meal and multiply it by 40%.

Calories per meal _256_ × 50% = _126_ Calories from protein for each meal

Because protein contains 4 calories per gram, divide the above number by 4 to determine the number of grams of protein per meal.

Protein calories per meal _126_ ÷ 4 = _31_ **Grams of protein per meal**

Now use the same formula to determine the fat content of each meal. Take the number of calories per meal and multiply it by 20%.

Calories per meal _256_ × 20% = _51_ Fat calories per meal

Now, because fat contains 9 calories per gram, take the number of fat calories per meal and divide it by 9—this will be the number of fat grams per meal.

Fat calories per meal _51_ ÷ 9 = _5_ **Grams of fat per meal**

Now let's summarize the figures.

- **Grams of carbohydrate per meal** _25_
- **Grams of protein per meal** _31_
- **Grams of fat per meal** _5_

PUTTING THE NUMBERS TO WORK

Now that you have successfully completed all the necessary calculations for the plan, its time to put them into action. Getting the right amounts of the different food groups is very important, so take your time and make sure you fully understand. You may need to read this part of the chapter two times, but once you really understand all these numbers, you will be equipped to have great success.

Portion Sizes

Determining your portion sizes is fairly easy, it just takes a couple of simple steps. Simply take the number of grams of carbohydrate, protein, or fat you need per meal, and divide it by the number of grams of carbohydrate per portion listed on the food list. Please examine the examples that appear on the following page.

Example #1

Let's say that you need 21 grams of protein per meal. You have chosen to have fish. Fish contains, on average, 7 grams of protein per oz., so you would have 3 oz. (21 grams protein ÷ 7 grams protein/oz. = 3 oz.).

Example #2

If you needed 40 grams of carbohydrate per meal, and you chose to eat yams, you would have about 6 oz., because cooked yams contain about 7 grams carbohydrate per oz. (40 grams carbohydrate ÷ 7 grams carbohydrate in an oz. = about 6 oz.).

All amounts listed on the food list are after cooking, except oatmeal, which is measured prior to cooking. I highly recommend that you weigh your portions a few times to become familiar with what amounts you should be eating. After just a few times weighing these foods, you will be able to "eyeball" the amounts.

If you do not see a particular food that you want to eat on the list, avoid that food for the first month. After that, simply determine how much carbohydrate, protein and fat the food contains, and calculate how much you need to have. Remember though—avoid all non-listed foods for the first month.

Table 16.01

40/40/20 Plan Food List

PROTEINS	CARBOHYDRATES	FATS

PROTEINS

Chicken breast*

Turkey breast*

Venison*

Beefalo*

Buffalo*

Fish*

Shellfish*

Lamb

Veal

7% fat ground beef

Lean steaks

Lean cuts of pork

Canadian bacon

Ham
Average 7 grams protein/oz.

Egg whites*
3 grams protein each

Egg substitute*
Check label for protein content.

Nonfat cottage cheese *Average 3 grams protein/oz.*

Nonfat cheese
Average 9 grams protein/oz.

Tofu/Soy protein products
Check label for protein content. Watch for extra carbs and fats.

Protein powders*
Microfiltered, ion-exchanged, predigested **whey** *protein is best.*

CARBOHYDRATES

Yams/Sweet potatoes*

Red potatoes*
7 grams carbohydrate/oz.

Rice* 2/3c
37 grams carbohydrate/cup

Oats* 1/3c
27 grams carbohydrate 1/2 cup—uncooked

Beans/Lentils* 2/3c
Average 35 grams carbohydrate/cup

Breads
Check label for carbohydrate content.

Bagels 1/2 bagel
Average 50 carbohydrates per bagel—check label.

Corn tortillas
Average 12 carbohydrates each

Flour tortillas
Average 20 carbohydrates each—check label.

Fruit 1 small fruit
Average 35 carbohydrates per small piece

Melon
Average 45 carbohydrates per melon

Pasta 2/3c
38 carbohydrates per cup

FATS

Safflower oil*

Sunflower oil*

Hemp oil*

Olive oil*

Canola oil*

Peanut oil*

Tahini oil*

Soybean oil*
Best not to cook oils 4 grams fat per tsp.

Nuts*
Check label for fat content.

Nut butters* 2tsp
Average 3 grams fat per tsp.

Avocado*
3 grams fat per tbsp.

Olives* 5-6
1 gram fat each

Seeds*
Average 12 grams fat/oz.

Butter 1/6 pat
9 grams fat per pat
14 grams fat per tbsp.

Mayonnaise < 1/2 tbsp
14 grams fat per tbsp.

Cream
5 grams fat per tbsp.

Cheese
Check label for fat content.

*Indicates best choices
All amounts listed are after cooking

Table 16.02

Free Foods List

The following foods are free foods. Unless otherwise noted, you can consume them at any time, with or without meals.

All vegetables *Except corn, peas, squash, carrots, beets*
Diet sodas *Avoid those containing phosphoric acid or caffeine or saccharin*
Diet flavored waters *Avoid those containing phosphoric acid or caffeine or saccharin*
Crystal Light
Regular coffee *Up to 2 cups per day*
Unlimited decaffeinated coffee *Preferably water processed*
Herbal teas *Caffeine-free*
Iced tea *Sugar-free; avoid saccharin; decaffeinated; green tea is best*
Swiss Miss diet cocoa *Up to 2 packets per day*
Sugar-free Jell-o
Sugar-free gum
Frozen yogurt *Maximum 4 oz., 2 times per week*
Gise Frozen Yogurt (800) 448-4473
Nonfat sour cream
Nonfat cream cheese
Nonfat mayonnaise
Nonfat salad dressing *Maximum of 2 tbsp. per day*
Citrus peels
Vinegars
Lemon and lime juice
Extracts
All dry seasonings and herbal seasonings
BBQ, Teriyaki, Mustard, Relish, Salsa, Ketchup, A-1,
Soy sauce (low sodium)

Note: Consumption of aspartame-containing food products is a personal decision. Much data exists to support its safety, but this continues to be a much-debated issue.

YOUR FIRST WEEK

It is an understatement to say that during your first week, your body will be going through significant changes. You will be bringing back balance to what may have been unbalanced for your entire life. You may have never in your life arrived at what is correct for you. During this first week, you will be rearranging the levels of hormones that make up the metabolism. As a result, you may be feeling certain things that are unusual for you. You may be depressed, or you may feel euphoric. You may get some acne, or you may eliminate the acne that you have. Your energy may soar, keeping you up at night, or you may feel totally lethargic for the first week. You will go through a number of metabolic changes that will result in symptoms that I am not able to predict.

What you must do is keep going forward, no matter what. I liken this to the way you would drive a car. You place your foot on the gas pedal, and the car begins to move forward. If you hold the gas pedal down, the car travels faster and faster. As the car travels faster, it also uses up more fuel. This fuel consumption allows the car to travel even faster. What happens when you let your foot off the gas pedal? The car slows back down. In other words, if you deprive yourself of food, you will not have enough gas in your engine. If you feel like you are eating too much, or change the way you should be eating because you are feeling a certain way, *you will never get over the hump*. You will never reach freeway speeds, and you will be stuck on side-streets forever. So keep going forward no matter what. For this first week you will have to go on faith. Don't let up, and you will be well on your journey.

HELPFUL HINTS

You must not miss meals. If you do not eat **four** times a day at least 80% of the time, you will not succeed.

If you happen to overeat one meal, do **not** *undereat during the next meal*. In other words, do not alter any meal, based on a mistake you made on the meal prior to that, or in anticipation of a meal that is ahead of you. By doing this you will have ruined *two* meals. Each meal is its own separate entity, and is not reliant on any other meal. Each meal is like taking a medicine that we are trying to get an effect from, that will wear off in a few hours, so we would take that medicine again. If you change the medicine once, would you change the medicine again to account for that? No. You can't double up, you can't cut it in half. You will simply be ruining a half of your day instead of a quarter of your day. Even in cases of extreme overeating, the next meal is exactly as it should be. We are attempting to create an environment for your metabolism. Allow that environment to be as stable as possible. The same applies to undereating. Do not eat more the next time.

You've heard it a hundred times, but I'll say it again. You must drink enough water. If you are dehydrated, you will not burn fat. End of story. Water is necessary in the process of not only fat reduction, but every metabolic process. If you are not drinking enough water, you will fail. You should be urinating about ten times per day for your fat to remove itself from your body. If you are not in the bathroom more than you think you should be, you are not in there enough. Drink at least eight 12-oz. glasses of water each day.

Purchase a food scale. Don't assume that you know anything, even if you have been on a program where you had to weigh your food. It is vital that you are getting the proper amount of food in the correct ratios for this to work for you. You don't want to be, and you don't need to be measuring everything that you eat. However, for the first week or so, I want you to get a better idea of what your portion size will look like. If you have determined, by using "The Perfect Portion," that you need 6 oz. of protein with each meal, weigh that out before and after cooking. Put it in your bowl of salad or on the plate, so that you can be accustomed to what that portion size looks like. Give yourself that edge, you'll thank me for it down the road. If you are unable to locate a scale, call toll-free (888) 663-2881.

For this or any other plan, preparation is key. Know that if you will be in the middle of nowhere when mealtime rolls around, that you will have brought something to eat with you. If you know that you will be in the middle of a meeting when mealtime comes around, bring a meal replacement in with you, so that you do not activate your starvation protection mechanism. You don't have to eat a meal, you just have to ingest the proper amounts of carbohy-drate, protein and fat. Prepare a thermos full of a meal replacement drink, to have throughout the day. Don't go out into the world everyday, and just expect that the right food will be there. It won't be there. Think ahead. Plan for your success.

Make sure you are getting enough protein. Most menu items will not have the necessary protein content. You must learn to order additional portions, or let them know exactly how much you need. You must make an Olympian effort to get enough protein.

Foods must be eaten together at the same time to bring about the desired results. A major point of eating in this prescribed man-ner is to stimulate or repress the production of specific hormones that make up the metabolism. To foster this hormone activity, these foods must be ingested as a whole. Do not, under any cir-cumstances, have a protein without the fat portion of the meal or vice versa. These food groups will always be consumed at the same time, or eating will have the exact opposite outcome than the results you desire.

Do not have more than two alcoholic beverages per week. If you have a couple (two) glasses of alcohol per week, it should have no effect. Your body will absorb it, and you won't even see it. Any greater alcohol consumption and it is a ball and chain wrapped around your waist that you are dragging with you 24 hours a day. The alcoholic portion of any beverage you consume *will* be con-verted to body-fat. For women this body-fat is gathered at the back of the arms, the hips and just below the belly button. For men, it seems to gather between the chest and the pelvic area.

It is most beneficial to have vegetables with each meal. Vegetables will not only eliminate any trace of carbohydrate crav-ing, but will also be very filling, and regulate the bowels very suc-cessfully. In addition to these benefits, many vegetables are high in the EFAs and contain special nutrients that are tremendously bene-ficial to the human body.

The correct supplementation program can dramatically enhance your results. My experience with thousands of clients has proven that the proper diet combined with a well-designed supple-mentation program will provide an average of approximately *30% increased rate of fat reduction*. In addition to faster and greater fat reduction, you can achieve a stronger immune system, higher energy levels, and most importantly a higher success rate of maintenance. You will find a comprehensive guide to these supplements in Chapter 5.

Meal replacement "Protein bars" are an excellent way to have a meal in a hurry or on-the-go. Depending on which plan you have chosen, you will be required to eat 4–7 times per day. In many cases, this is a difficult task, one that can be made much easier with the option of having a meal replacement bar. Just open the wrapper and eat your meal—it is as easy as that. You can use these bars as often as needed, as long as they contain the appropriate amounts of proteins, carbohydrates, and fats. There are many of these bars available. The trick is to find the bar that contains the necessary amounts of proteins, carbohydrates, and fats for your plan. To find the right bar, just go to your local health food store and either look at the labels yourself, or ask for help. You can also call (888) 663-2881 to have some of the right bars sent to you.

**Finally, you have what it takes to get lean.
Now go for it!**

## 17

RECIPES & COOKING

*B*on Appetit!

In the past, "dieting" almost always meant that you would eat unappealing foods.

It doesn't have to be that way!

Foods can be prepared to offer the sophisticated pallet a plethora of taste sensations that enable you to look forward to eating, and eating well. In short, food that tastes great helps you to stick to the program of your choice, and in the end, succeed.

Now that you have determined the ideal plan to fit your needs, you may need some guidance for menu planning, or just get some new ideas about how to prepare food that tastes great and also fits within the parameters of your new nutritional plan. After determining portion sizes for each food group, you will have a much clearer idea of how much of each of these foods you should have.

As you browse through this chapter, you will notice that at the bottom of each recipe are notations indicating which programs that recipe applies to, and the nutritional value of the dish. The recipes will serve as a helpful outline to make a great meal, but the differing needs of the individual require your participation, and may require you to do some simple calculations.

SOUPS

SPRING GREENS SOUP

2 teaspoons olive oil
3 green onions, chopped
¾ cup shredded spinach
¾ cup shredded butter lettuce
¾ cup chopped watercress
3 tablespoons chopped flat-leaf parsley
3 cups chicken stock or low-fat broth
2 tablespoons plain yogurt and
2 tablespoons low-fat sour cream
salt and freshly ground black pepper
chopped chives

In a saucepan, heat the oil and sauté the onions until tender. Add the greens and parsley; cover and steam 5 minutes. Add the stock and simmer 10 minutes. Stir in the yogurt and sour cream. Season with salt and pepper. Puree in a blender or food processor.

This Recipe Will Work With:

- Super EFA
- 3+2
- Insulin Buster
- Protein Plus One
- 30/50/20
- 50/30/20
- 40/40/20
- Unlimited Protein & Vegetables

This entire recipe contains 10 grams of fat. Use the appropriate amount of soup to fulfill the fat requirements for a given meal. All other ingredients are free foods.

COOL CUCUMBER SOUP

4 hothouse cucumbers
1 container (16 ounces) plain nonfat sour cream
1 can (14 ounces) chicken broth
1 medium shallot, minced
1 medium-sized dill pickle
¼ cup pickle juice
2 tablespoons fresh dill
1 teaspoon salt
1 teaspoon lemon zest
nonfat sour cream, fresh dill, and a dollop of
    salmon caviar for garnish

In large bowl, combine all ingredients except garnish. In food processor with knife blade attached, blend half of cucumber mixture just until cucumbers are finely chopped but not pureed. Pour mixture into soup tureen. Repeat with remaining cucumber mixture; add to soup in tureen. Refrigerate soup if not serving right away. To serve, garnish each bowl of soup with some caviar and dill sprig.

This Recipe Will Work With:

- Super EFA
- 3+2
- Protein Plus One
- 30/50/20
- 50/30/20
- 40/40/20
- Unlimited Protein & Vegetables

This is a free food for the above plans.

ZUCCHINI SOUP

3 pounds zucchini
4 cups chopped onion
3 cups chicken broth
1 clove garlic, minced
3 tablespoons curry powder
salt and pepper to taste
2 cups low-fat sour cream
1 cup chopped green onions

Chop zucchini into 1-inch cubes and set aside. To a non-stick sauce pan, add chopped onion. Cook, stirring until onion is wilted. Add zucchini and curry powder and cook a minute or two longer. Add chicken broth, garlic, and salt and pepper to taste. Cover and simmer for 5 minutes. Remove from heat and chill. Stir in low-fat sour cream. Garnish with chopped green onions.

This Recipe Will Work With:

- Super EFA
- 3+2
- Protein Plus One
- 30/50/20
- 50/30/20
- 40/40/20
- Unlimited Protein & Vegetables

This is a free food for the above plans.

GAZPACHO WITH CILANTRO CREAM

2 medium cucumbers, peeled
1 medium yellow pepper
¼ small red onion
1 pound ripe tomatoes, peeled, seeded
1 small jalapeño chili, seeded
3 tablespoons fresh lime juice
1 teaspoon extra virgin olive oil
1 cup tomato juice
salt to taste
¼ cup non-fat sour cream
finely chopped cilantro

Chop red onions, cucumber, yellow pepper, tomatoes, and jalapeño. Add lime juice, olive oil, salt, and tomato juice. Cover and refrigerate until well chilled. In small bowl, mix sour cream, 4 teaspoons chopped cilantro, and pinch salt. Serve cold soup with cilantro cream.

This Recipe Will Work With:

- 3+2
- Protein Plus One
- 30/50/20
- 50/30/20
- 40/40/20
- Unlimited Protein & Vegetables

This is a free food for the above plans.

MUSSEL SOUP

2 pounds small mussels, scrubbed with
   beards removed
1 tablespoon olive oil
1 large onion, sliced
2 garlic cloves, minced
1 28-ounce can plum tomatoes in puree
1 8-ounce bottle clam juice
½ cup dry white wine
¼ teaspoon salt
⅛ teaspoon crushed red pepper
2 tablespoons chopped fresh parsley
green onions for garnish

In 5-quart Dutch oven, heat olive oil over medium heat. Add onion and cook until tender and lightly browned, about 10 minutes. Add garlic; cook 2 minutes longer. Stir in tomatoes with their puree, clam juice, white wine, salt, red pepper, and 2 cups water. Heat to boiling over high heat, stirring and breaking up tomatoes. Simmer to meld flavors for 20 minutes. Add mussels and simmer until all mussels are open about five minutes.

This Recipe Will Work With:

- Super EFA
- 3+2
- Protein Plus One
- 30/50/20
- 50/30/20
- 40/40/20
- Unlimited Protein & Vegetables

This entire recipe contains 200 grams of protein. This recipe contains approximately 20 grams of fat (1 gram of fat for every 10 grams of protein).

EGGPLANT-TOMATO BISQUE

1 large onion, finely chopped
1 teaspoon olive oil
1 small eggplant
1 cup pureed plum tomatoes
3 cups low-fat chicken broth
salt and pepper to taste
2 garlic cloves, minced
freshly chopped basil

In a heavy saucepan, sauté the onion in oil until golden. Meanwhile, cut the eggplant into wedges, sprinkle with salt, and let stand 15 minutes for the juices to exude. Rinse, peel, and chop. Add the eggplant to the onions along with the tomatoes, chicken broth, salt, pepper, and garlic. Cover and simmer 10 minutes, or until the eggplant is tender. Puree in a blender or food processor. Return to the pan and reheat. Ladle into bowls and garnish with basil.

This Recipe Will Work With:

- Super EFA
- 3+2
- Protein Plus One
- 30/50/20
- 50/30/20
- 40/40/20
- Unlimited Protein & Vegetables

This is a free food for the above plans.

POULTRY

ROASTED TURKEY BREAST WITH SALSA

> 1 turkey breast (about 3 to 4 pounds)
> salt and freshly ground pepper
> 3 garlic cloves, slivered
> 1 lemon, halved

Season the turkey with salt and pepper and lemon juice. Place in a 350-degree pre-heated oven and bake 15 to 20 minutes per pound of turkey.

Mexican Salsa

> 4 tomatoes, peeled and diced
> 3 green onions, chopped
> ¼ cup chopped Italian parsley
> 3 tablespoons chopped fresh cilantro
> 1 garlic clove, minced
> 2 tablespoons diced canned green chili pepper
>   or fresh hot pepper
> salt and freshly ground black pepper

Combine all ingredients in a large bowl and mix well. Cover and chill several hours.

This Recipe Will Work With:

- 3+2
- Protein Plus One
- 30/50/20
- 50/30/20
- 40/40/20
- Unlimited Protein & Vegetables

Cooked turkey yields 7 grams of protein per ounce. The salsa is a free food for the above plans.

ORIENTAL CHICKEN SALAD

2 ounces Jicama
the appropriate amount of chicken torn in strips
8 ounces iceberg lettuce, finely sliced
2 tablespoons red ginger, sliced
4 ounces blanched bean sprouts
1 green onion, sliced diagonally and finely
⅛ cup toasted peanuts
fresh cilantro

Cook chicken in chicken broth until done. Tear into strips, squeeze out liquid and add to all other ingredients. Serve with ¼ cup dressing.

Dressing

¾ cup soy sauce
¼ cup seasoned rice vinegar
4 tablespoons dark sesame oil
1 teaspoon salt
1 teaspoon Sambal red pepper sauce
julienne of fresh ginger

This Recipe Will Work With:

- 3+2
- Protein Plus One
- 30/50/20
- 50/30/20
- 40/40/20
- Unlimited Protein & Vegetables

The dressing for this salad counts as a fat for the above plans, and yields 3 grams of fat per teaspoon. The amount of protein is determined by the amount of chicken used.

INDONESIAN CHICKEN SATAY

1½ pounds boneless chicken breast
1 medium onion, chopped
4 teaspoons freshly ground coriander seeds
dash cayenne
1½ tablespoons brown sugar
2 garlic cloves, minced
salt and freshly ground black pepper to taste
3 tablespoons lemon juice
¼ cup soy sauce
satay sauce (recipe follows)

Cut the meat into 1-inch cubes. Place in a mixing bowl the onion, coriander, cayenne, sugar, garlic, salt, pepper, lemon juice, and soy; mix well. Add the meat, stir to coat, cover, and chill for several hours. Thread the meat on skewers and broil or barbecue over medium coals until cooked through. Can be served with or without satay sauce.

This Recipe Will Work With:

- Super EFA
- 3+2
- Insulin Buster
- Protein Plus One
- Hi/Lo
- 7-Day Quick Fix
- 30/50/20
- 50/30/20
- 40/40/20
- Unlimited Protein & Vegetables

This portion of the recipe (no sauce) counts as a protein for the above plans. The entire recipe yields 150 grams of protein.

SATAY SAUCE

¼ teaspoon ground cumin
¼ teaspoon ground coriander
¼ teaspoon ground turmeric
¼ teaspoon pepper
1 teaspoon butter
2 tablespoons peanut butter
1 teaspoon lemon juice
¼ cup water
1 teaspoon brown sugar
1 garlic clove, minced
1 tablespoon chopped shallots or green onion
salt and liquid hot pepper seasoning to taste

Sauté cumin, coriander, turmeric, and pepper in butter for one to two minutes, stirring constantly. Add peanut butter, lemon juice, water, brown sugar, garlic, and shallots or green onion. Season with salt and liquid hot pepper seasoning.

This Recipe Will Work With:

- Super EFA
- 3+2
- Insulin Buster
- Protein Plus One
- 30/50/20
- 50/30/20
- 40/40/20
- Unlimited Protein & Vegetables

This portion of the recipe counts as a fat. The entire recipe yields 15 grams of fat.

CHICKEN CHILI

2 teaspoons vegetable oil
4 cups coarsely chopped onion
1 cup coarsely chopped green pepper
4 cloves garlic, thinly sliced
1 pound ground chicken breast (95% fat-free)
¼ cup chili powder
1 teaspoon ground cumin
2 teaspoon ground coriander
1 teaspoon salt
1 teaspoon cayenne pepper
2 (14 oz.) cans no-salt-added tomatoes, undrained
   and chopped
2 (10 oz.) cans low-salt chicken broth
1 bay leaf
beans

In a Teflon-lined saucepan add oil. Add onion, bell pepper, garlic; sauté 5 minutes. Add chicken and cook 10 minutes or until browned, stirring constantly. Add chili powder, ground cumin, coriander, salt, and cayenne. Cook 1 minute, stirring constantly. Add chopped tomatoes, broth, and bay leaf. Cover, reduce heat, simmer 40 minutes, stirring occasionally. Add appropriate amount of beans per your menu plan; cook, uncovered, an additional 20 minutes, stirring occasionally. Discard bay leaf.

This Recipe Will Work With:

- Super EFA
- 3+2
- Insulin Buster
- Protein Plus One
- Hi/Lo
- 7-Day Quick Fix
- 30/50/20
- 50/30/20
- 40/40/20
- Unlimited Protein & Vegetables

This recipe counts as a protein for the above plans. The entire recipe yields 150 grams of protein.

GRILLED CHICKEN LETTUCE ROLL
WITH TOMATO AND BASIL

1 boneless, skinless chicken breast
granulated garlic
paprika
pinch of salt
sliced tomato
whole lettuce leaves
basil leaves
non-fat mayonnaise

Flatten chicken breast. Season with salt, granulated garlic, and paprika. Cook thoroughly on grill until opaque, about 10 minutes on each side. Slice chicken into 1-inch strips. Spread non-fat mayonnaise on one half of the lettuce. Add chicken breast, slice of tomato, and 2 or 3 basil leaves.

This Recipe Will Work With:

- Super EFA
- 3+2
- Insulin Buster
- Protein Plus One
- Hi/Lo
- 7-Day Quick Fix
- 30/50/20
- 50/30/20
- 40/40/20
- Unlimited Protein & Vegetables

This recipe counts as a protein for the above plans. The amount of protein is determined by the amount of chicken used.

MEATS

ROLLED LEG OF LAMB
WITH ROASTED GARLIC

1 head garlic
3 pounds boneless leg of lamb, rolled and tied
salt and freshly ground black pepper to taste
1 teaspoon olive oil

Preheat the oven to 325°F. Peel and sliver 2 or 3 garlic cloves and insert the slivers in the folds of the meat. Season the meat with salt and pepper and place it on a roasting pan. Insert a meat thermometer. Slice the papery wrapper from the top of the garlic head and drizzle it with oil. Wrap in foil. Roast the meat and garlic in the oven allowing about 45 minutes for the garlic and 50 to 55 minutes for the meat, or until the meat thermometer registers 145°F for rare meat or 160°F for medium meat. Let the meat stand a few minutes. Slice and serve each plate with a few cloves of garlic to squeeze over. Makes 10 servings.

This Recipe Will Work With:

- Super EFA
- 3+2
- Insulin Buster
- Protein Plus One
- 30/50/20
- 50/30/20
- 40/40/20
- Unlimited Protein & Vegetables

This recipe counts as a protein for the above plans. Each serving contains 30 grams of protein and 3 grams of fat.

SPICED BUTTERFLIED LAMB

1 cup plain low-fat sour cream
8 garlic cloves, peeled
1 piece fresh ginger (about 2 inches), peeled and
    coarsely chopped
1 tablespoon ground coriander
1 tablespoon ground cumin
2 tablespoons fresh lemon juice
2 teaspoons salt
½ teaspoon ground red pepper (cayenne)
3 pounds boneless butterflied leg of lamb

In blender, combine sour cream with remaining ingredients except lamb and blend until smooth. Pour this mixture over lamb and refrigerate 1 hour, turning. Remove lamb from marinade, saving marinade for later. Place lamb on grill over medium heat; cook 15 minutes, turning once. Brush both sides of lamb with reserved marinade and cook 10 to 20 minutes longer for medium rare or until it reaches desired doneness, turning lamb occasionally. The thickness of butterflied lamb will vary throughout; cut off sections of lamb as they are cooked and place on cutting board.

This Recipe Will Work With:

- Super EFA
- 3+2
- Insulin Buster
- Protein Plus One
- 30/50/20
- 50/30/20
- 40/40/20
- Unlimited Protein & Vegetables

This recipe counts as a protein for the above plans. The entire recipe yields 310 grams of protein, and 1 gram of fat for every 10 grams of protein.

KOREAN-STYLE STEAK

½ cup reduced-sodium soy sauce
2 tablespoons minced, peeled fresh ginger
2 tablespoons seasoned rice vinegar
1 tablespoon Asian sesame oil
¼ teaspoon ground red pepper (cayenne)
3 garlic cloves, crushed with garlic press
1 beef top round steak, 1 inch thick
3 green onions, thinly sliced
1 tablespoon sesame seeds, toasted
1 medium head romaine lettuce, separated into leaves
2 cups rice

In large self-sealing plastic bag, combine soy sauce, sugar, ginger, vinegar, sesame oil, ground red pepper, and garlic; add steak, turning to coat. Seal bag, pressing out excess air. Place bag on plate; refrigerate steak 1 to 4 hours to marinate, turning once.

Just before grilling steak, prepare rice as label directs; keep warm. Remove steak from bag; reserve marinade. Place steak on grill over medium heat and cook 14 to 15 minutes for medium rare or until it reaches desired doneness, turning steak once. Transfer steak to cutting board; let stand 10 minutes to allow juices to set for easier slicing. In 1-quart saucepan, heat reserved marinade and ¼ cup water to boiling over high heat; boil 2 minutes.

To serve, thinly slice steak. Let each person place some steak slices, rice, green onions, and sesame seeds on a lettuce leaf, then drizzle with some cooked marinade. Fold sides of lettuce leaf over filling to make a package to eat out of hand.

This Recipe Will Work With:

- Super EFA
- 3+2
- Insulin Buster
- Protein Plus One
- 30/50/20
- 50/30/20
- 40/40/20
- Unlimited Protein & Vegetables

This recipe counts as a protein for the above plans. This recipe yields 7 grams of protein and 2 grams of fat per ounce.

ROASTED STUFFED RED PEPPER

 12 red bell peppers
 1 pound extra lean ground beef
 1 cup finely chopped onions
 2 egg whites
 1 cup cooked rice
 1 teaspoon soy sauce
 1 teaspoon salt
 1 green onion
 4 cloves garlic
 ¼ teaspoon black pepper
 2 teaspoons sesame oil
 1 tablespoon crushed sesame seeds

Halve the red peppers and remove seeds. Sauté onions in a nonstick pan until transparent. Add the ground beef and sauté well. Mix the ground beef, cooked rice, egg whites, soy, green onions, garlic and seasonings. Stuff the pepper halves with the beef mixture. Place in baking dish. Garnish with the sesame seeds and bake at 325 degrees for 1 hour. Can also be garnished with tomato sauce.

This Recipe Will Work With:

- Super EFA
- 3+2
- Insulin Buster
- Protein Plus One
- 30/50/20
- 50/30/20
- 40/40/20
- Unlimited Protein & Vegetables

This recipe yields 9 grams of protein and 5 grams of carbohydrate per pepper.

SLICED TRI-TIP STEAK

1 tritip beef roast approximately 3 pounds
granulated garlic
paprika, salt, black pepper to taste

Trim excess fat from meat. Rub spice well into tri-tip.
Barbecue on grill, 15 minutes on each side until done
medium rare. Let rest 10 minutes after cooking. Slice
thinly across the grain and serve. Excellent hot or cold, or
in salads.

This Recipe Will Work With:

- Super EFA
- 3+2
- Insulin Buster
- Protein Plus One
- 30/50/20
- 50/30/20
- 40/40/20
- Unlimited Protein & Vegetables

This recipe counts as a protein for the above plans. Cooked
(de-fatted) tri-tip yields 7 grams of protein and 1 gram of
fat per ounce.

ROAST BEEF SALAD

1 cup broccoli florets
1 cup mixed baby greens
4 ounces cooked roast tri-tip, cut into thin strips
2 thin slices red onion
1 thin sliced cucumber
1 tomato, quartered
1 tablespoon chopped fresh mint
1 teaspoon peanut oil
juice of 1 lime
red pepper flakes

Combine all ingredients and serve.

This Recipe Will Work With:

- 3+2
- Insulin Buster
- Protein Plus One
- 30/50/20
- 50/30/20
- 40/40/20
- Unlimited Protein & Vegetables

This recipe counts as a protein for the above plans. Cooked (de-fatted) tri-tip yields 7 grams of protein and 1 gram of fat per ounce.

FISH AND SEAFOOD

UNFRIED RED SNAPPER

four red snapper filets
¼ cup soy sauce
three chopped scallions
four tablespoons minced ginger root
1 teaspoon lemon zest
1 tablespoon sesame oil

Simmer each filet in lightly salted water until tender, being careful not to overcook. Drain, arrange on serving plate. Sprinkle with soy sauce, scallions, lemon zest, and ginger. Heat oil carefully until boiling, and pour over fish. Serve immediately.

This Recipe Will Work With:

- Super EFA
- 3+2
- Insulin Buster
- Protein Plus One
- Hi/Lo
- 7-Day Quick Fix
- 30/50/20
- 50/30/20
- 40/40/20
- Unlimited Protein & Vegetables

This recipe counts as a protein for the above plans. The amount of protein is determined by the amount of fish eaten. For the "Hi/Lo" and "7-Day Quick Fix," delete oil from recipe.

AHI (TUNA) BURGERS

1 pound tuna steak
1 green onion, diagonally finely sliced
2 tablespoons low sodium soy sauce
1 teaspoon grated fresh ginger
¼ teaspoon coarsely ground black pepper
1 egg white

Finely chop tuna with a knife. Mix in green onion, soy sauce, ginger, egg white, and pepper. Shape tuna mixture into four patties. Place tuna patties on nonstick pan over medium heat and cook 6 to 7 minutes, until browned on the outside and still slightly pink in the center, turning patties over once.

This Recipe Will Work With:

- Super EFA
- 3+2
- Insulin Buster
- Protein Plus One
- Hi/Lo
- 7-Day Quick Fix
- 30/50/20
- 50/30/20
- 40/40/20
- Unlimited Protein & Vegetables

This recipe counts as a protein for the above plans. This recipe yields 25 grams of protein per patty.

SEAFOOD SKEWERS WITH LIME AND DILL

8 ounces large ocean scallops
8 ounces medium-size shrimp
8 ounces (1-inch) cubes sea bass or halibut fillet
⅓ cup fresh lime juice
1 large clove garlic, minced
1 tablespoon black sesame oil
2 tablespoons chopped fresh dill
6 cherry tomatoes
6 fresh white mushrooms
12 pearl onions
brown rice

Mix lime juice, fresh garlic, chopped dill, and sesame oil. Marinate all the seafood, mushrooms, tomatoes, and pearl onions in this mixture for 2 hours in refrigerator. Skewer seafood and vegetables and secure with pearl onions on each end. Grill lightly for about 4 minutes on each side. Brush with marinade while grilling. Serve over brown rice.

This Recipe Will Work With:

- Super EFA
- 3+2
- Insulin Buster
- Protein Plus One
- Hi/Lo
- 7-Day Quick Fix
- 30/50/20
- 50/30/20
- 40/40/20
- Unlimited Protein & Vegetables

This recipe counts as a protein for the above plans. The entire recipe contains 150 grams of protein. Simply delete sesame oil for the "Hi/Lo" and "7-Day Quick Fix."

MUSSELS WITH SAFFRON TOMATO BROTH

4 pounds mussels, scrubbed well
2 bay leaves
large pinch of saffron
1 tablespoon olive oil
1 cup onion, chopped
2 cloves crushed garlic
2 cups chopped plum tomatoes
2 cups clam or chicken broth
2 tablespoon freshly chopped coriander
1 teaspoon salt

In a large stock pan place cleaned mussels and bay leaves without water cover and steam until all mussels open. Discard any that do not open. Save all mussel liquid. Meanwhile, sauté onions, garlic, and saffron in olive oil. Add tomatoes and broth, and cook for 10 minutes over medium heat. Pour over mussels and mussel liquid. Season with salt and garnish with coriander.

This Recipe Will Work With:

- Super EFA
- 3+2
- Insulin Buster
- Protein Plus One
- Hi/Lo
- 7-Day Quick Fix
- 30/50/20
- 50/30/20
- 40/40/20
- Unlimited Protein & Vegetables

This recipe counts as a protein for the above plans. The entire recipe contains 400 grams of protein. Simply delete olive oil for the "Hi/Lo" and "7-Day Quick Fix."

SWORDFISH WITH ORANGE SOY

2 (4-ounce) swordfish steaks, 1 inch thick
1 teaspoon olive oil
3 tablespoons finely grated zest of orange
1 tablespoon low-sodium soy sauce
1 cup chopped ripe tomato
2 tablespoons capers, drained
parsley

Heat a large nonstick frying pan; add 1 teaspoon olive oil and the swordfish steaks. Grill 3 minutes on each side. Remove to a heated platter. Add tomatoes capers and soy, and cook 3 minutes. Add the orange zest and garnish with parsley and orange slices. Serve at once.

This Recipe Will Work With:

- Super EFA
- 3+2
- Insulin Buster
- Protein Plus One
- 30/50/20
- 50/30/20
- 40/40/20
- Unlimited Protein & Vegetables

This recipe counts as protein for the above plans. The entire recipe contains 50 grams of protein.

BOUILLABAISSE

2 pounds boneless Chilean sea bass or halibut
1 pound sea scallops
1 pound cleaned large shrimp
1 dozen live clams
1 dozen medium-size live black mussels
3 medium-sized chopped onions
3 cups grated fresh fennel
2 teaspoon olive oil
2 garlic cloves, minced
4 cups clam juice or chicken broth
1 teaspoon white pepper
1 teaspoon saffron threads
2 tablespoons chopped parsley

Cut fish into 1-inch pieces. Slice horizontally each scallop in half. In a large saucepan place clams and mussels, cover and heat until shells just open, about 5 minutes. In another large nonstick saucepan over medium heat, cook olive oil, saffron, onions, garlic, and fennel until tender, about 15 minutes. Add fish. Reduce heat to medium-low; cook uncovered, 5 to 8 minutes. Add shrimp and scallops and cook for 2 minutes. Add clams and mussels and sprinkle with parsley.

This Recipe Will Work With:

- Super EFA
- 3+2
- Insulin Buster
- Protein Plus One
- Hi/Lo
- 7-Day Quick Fix
- 30/50/20
- 50/30/20
- 40/40/20
- Unlimited Protein & Vegetables

This recipe counts as a protein for the above plans. The entire recipe yields 535 grams of protein. Simply delete oil for "Hi/Lo" and "7-Day Quick Fix."

CEVICHE

1 cup whitefish in 3/8" cubes
1 cup bay scallops
1 cup small shrimp
1 cup lemon juice
1 cup lime juice
1 bunch cilantro, chopped
1 cup chopped fresh tomatoes
1 chopped red onion
1 hot green chili, finely chopped
1 clove crushed garlic
1 teaspoon ground cumin
salt, pepper to taste
2 cups lettuce shredded
lime wedges
black olives for garnish

Marinate fresh fish, scallops, and shrimp in lemon-lime juice combination for 1 hour. Add cilantro, tomatoes, red onion, chili, garlic, olive oil, salt, and pepper. Refrigerate for at least 8 hours. Serve well chilled. Hand chop only, do not use processor.

This Recipe Will Work With:

- Super EFA
- 3+2
- Protein Plus One
- 30/50/20
- 50/30/20
- 40/40/20
- Unlimited Protein & Vegetables

Counts as a protein for the above plans. The entire recipe contains 160 grams of protein.

GINGER AND SOY WHOLE STEAMED FISH

> 1 whole rock cod or red snapper,
>   about 1 ¾ pounds
> 2 green onions
> 1 tablespoon light soy sauce
> 2 teaspoons dark sesame oil
> 1 tablespoon minced fresh ginger
> cilantro sprigs and green onion top "fans" for garnish

Rinse the fish and pat dry. Place on a heat-proof platter.
Chop the white part of the green onions diagonally into 1-
inch lengths and set these aside. Mix together the soy,
sesame oil, and ginger and set aside. Place the platter of
fish on a rack, pour over the sauce, and strew the chopped
onion on top. Cover and steam for 15 minutes or until the
fish is just opaque and firm to touch. Garnish with the
cilantro and green onion and serve the fish whole. At the
table, peel back the skin, and fillet the fish from the bones
to serve.

This Recipe Will Work With:

- Super EFA
- 3+2
- Insulin Buster
- Protein Plus One
- Hi/Lo
- 7-Day Quick Fix
- 30/50/20
- 50/30/20
- 40/40/20
- Unlimited Protein & Vegetables

This recipe counts as a protein for the above plans. The
amount of protein is determined by the amount of fish
eaten. Simply delete oil for the "Hi/Lo" and "7-Day
Quick-Fix."

SAUCES

SHRIMP COCKTAIL SAUCE

⅓ cup chili sauce
2 tablespoons lemon juice
1 tablespoon prepared horseradish
1 teaspoon Worcestershire sauce
dash of tabasco

Combine ingredients and chill thoroughly. Serve with boiled shrimp or cracked crab claws.

This Recipe Will Work With:

- Super EFA
- 3+2
- Insulin Buster
- Protein Plus One
- Hi/Lo
- 7-Day Quick Fix
- 30/50/20
- 50/30/20
- 40/40/20
- Unlimited Protein & Vegetables

This is a free food for all plans.

LOW FAT SALSA

3 ripe tomatoes, hand chopped
2 red or mild onions
1 bunch cilantro
green and red chilies to taste
dash of lemon juice
dash of olive oil
salt to taste

Combine all ingredients and serve.

This Recipe Will Work With:

- Super EFA
- 3+2
- Protein Plus One
- 30/50/20
- 50/30/20
- 40/40/20
- Unlimited Protein & Vegetables

This recipe is a free food for the above plans.

JAPANESE SALAD DRESSING

1 cup soy sauce (light, Kikkoman's)
¼ cup seasoned rice wine vinegar
1 tablespoon sesame oil (dark, oriental kind)
1 teaspoon grated ginger
1 teaspoon (or less) wasabe powder
   (green horseradish powder)

Mix ingredients well and chill.

This Recipe Will Work With:

- Super EFA
- 3+2
- Insulin Buster
- Protein Plus One
- 30/50/20
- 50/30/20
- 40/40/20
- Unlimited Protein & Vegetables

This recipe counts as a fat, and will yield approximately 1 gram of fat per teaspoon.

CAPER SAFFRON MAYONNAISE

1 tablespoon water
1 teaspoon packed saffron threads
¾ cup mayonnaise
¼ cup drained capers plus 1 teaspoon caper liquid
2 tablespoons mixed chopped fresh herbs (such as
    thyme, oregano, and parsley)
2 teaspoons fresh lemon juice
1 teaspoon minced garlic

Bring water and saffron to simmer in small saucepan. Remove from heat; let stand 10 minutes. Place mayonnaise in small bowl; whisk in saffron mixture. Add remaining ingredients; stir until blended. Season with salt and pepper. Cover and chill at least 2 hours.

This Recipe Will Work With:

- Super EFA
- 3+2
- Insulin Buster
- Protein Plus One
- 30/50/20
- 50/30/20
- 40/40/20
- Unlimited Protein & Vegetables

This recipe counts as a fat for the above plans. This recipe will yield approximately 2 grams of fat per teaspoon.

HERB BUTTER RECIPE (COMPOUND BUTTER)

> 1 pound butter
> 4 tablespoons finely chopped rosemary
> 8 tablespoons chopped parsley
> 2 tablespoons chopped garlic

Mix garlic and herbs with softened butter and roll into sausage shape in wax paper. Chill well. Slice ½" thick and garnish plate with 1 slice.

This Recipe Will Work With:

- Super EFA
- 3+2
- Insulin Buster
- Protein Plus One
- 30/50/20
- 50/30/20
- 40/40/20
- Unlimited Protein & Vegetables

This recipe counts as a fat for the above plans. This recipe will yield approximately 2.5 grams of fat per teaspoon.

RUTH'S ORIGINAL SAUCE

1 pint tahini (Middle Eastern brand)
1 quart mayonnaise
3 teaspoons red pepper, crushed
2 teaspoons crushed garlic
1 cup green onions, chopped
1 tablespoon lemon juice
¼ cup parsley
1 ¼ cups water

Combine all ingredients and chill well.

This Recipe Will Work With:

- Super EFA
- 3+2
- Insulin Buster
- Protein Plus One
- 30/50/20
- 50/30/20
- 40/40/20
- Unlimited Protein & Vegetables

This recipe counts as a fat for the above plans. This recipe will yield approximately 2 grams of fat per teaspoon.

TARTAR SAUCE

1 cup mayonnaise
2 tablespoons chopped gherkin pickles
2 tablespoons chopped capers
1 teaspoon chopped chives
1 teaspoon tarragon
¼ teaspoon chervil
¼ teaspoon dry mustard powder
2 teaspoons anchovy sauce

Put all ingredients into a bowl and mix thoroughly. Allow to stand for at least 30 minutes—this allows the flavors to meld.

This Recipe Will Work With:

- Super EFA
- 3+2
- Insulin Buster
- Protein Plus One
- 30/50/20
- 50/30/20
- 40/40/20
- Unlimited Protein & Vegetables

This recipe counts as a fat for the above plans. This recipe will yield approximately 2 grams of fat per teaspoon.

ORANGE TARRAGON BUTTER

½ cup (1 stick) butter, softened
2 teaspoons tarragon leaves, crushed
1 teaspoon grated orange peel
1 teaspoon salt
½ teaspoon ground black pepper

Place all ingredients in medium bowl; combine well and chill. Serve with hot cooked corn on the cob or other steamed vegetables.

This Recipe Will Work With:

- Super EFA
- 3+2
- Insulin Buster
- Protein Plus One
- 30/50/20
- 50/30/20
- 40/40/20
- Unlimited Protein & Vegetables

This recipe counts as a fat for the above plans. This recipe will yield approximately 2 grams of fat per teaspoon.

THAI PEANUT SAUCE

1 sliced small onion
1 tablespoon olive oil
¼ teaspoon cayenne
1 tablespoon soy sauce
1 teaspoon sugar
2 cloves crushed garlic
1 cup dry roasted salted peanuts
¼ teaspoon ground ginger
1 teaspoon salt
2 tablespoons lime juice

Sauté onion and garlic in oil until tender, cool. Place in blender, add everything else, and blend carefully. Slowly and carefully add enough boiling water to form a thick paste.

This Recipe Will Work With:

- Super EFA
- 3+2
- Insulin Buster
- Protein Plus One
- 30/50/20
- 50/30/20
- 40/40/20
- Unlimited Protein & Vegetables

This recipe counts as a fat for the above plans. This recipe will yield approximately 2.5 grams of fat per teaspoon.

SPICY CILANTRO BUTTER

4 cloves minced garlic
4 generous tablespoons chopped fresh cilantro
2 jalapeno peppers or 1 serrano chili, seeded
    and finely chopped
1 teaspoon lime zest (peel)
2–3 teaspoons fresh lime juice
salt to taste
crushed dried red chili to taste
¼ pound softened unsalted butter (one stick)

Blend all together. Good with grilled or broiled fish, shrimp, steak, pasta, rice, squash, corn, and eggplant. Roll corn on the cob in the butter, then sprinkle with Parmesan and lime juice.

This Recipe Will Work With:

- Super EFA
- 3+2
- Insulin Buster
- Protein Plus One
- 30/50/20
- 50/30/20
- 40/40/20
- Unlimited Protein & Vegetables

This recipe counts as a fat for the above plans. This recipe will yield approximately 3 grams of fat per teaspoon.

VEGETABLES

ORANGE, CUCUMBER, AND JICAMA SALAD

1 large head romaine
2 navel oranges, peeled and thinly sliced
1 cucumber, peeled and sliced
1 small red onion, sliced into rings
¾ cup peeled and chopped jicama
1 small red pepper, seeded, de-ribbed, and diced
2 tablespoons lemon juice
salt and freshly ground pepper

Tear the romaine into bite-sized pieces and place in a salad bowl. Arrange the oranges, cucumber, onion, jicama, and pepper on top. Mix together the lemon juice, salt, and pepper. Pour this dressing over the salad and mix lightly.

This Recipe Will Work With:

- Super EFA
- 3+2
- Insulin Buster
- Protein Plus One
- 30/50/20
- 50/30/20
- 40/40/20
- Unlimited Protein & Vegetables

This recipe counts as a free food for the above plans.

SWEET BUTTERNUT SQUASH

1 pound cooked butternut squash (peeled)
1 teaspoon cinnamon
1 teaspoon of nutmeg
2 teaspoons Equal sweetener

Mix all ingredients together in a bowl.

This Recipe Will Work With:

- Super EFA
- 3+2
- Insulin Buster
- Protein Plus One
- Hi/Lo
- 30/50/20
- 50/30/20
- 40/40/20
- Unlimited Protein & Vegetable

This recipe counts as a free food for the above plans. This recipe works with the "Hi/Lo" and the "7-Day Quick-Fix," but must be portioned appropriately.

CUCUMBER SALAD

3 cucumbers, medium sliced
1 cup white wine vinegar
3 teaspoons lemon juice
1 cup thinly sliced scallions
2 teaspoons Equal sweetener

Mix in a bowl, cover, and chill.

This Recipe Will Work With:

- Super EFA
- 3+2
- Insulin Buster
- Protein Plus One
- Hi/Lo
- 7-Day Quick Fix
- 30/50/20
- 50/30/20
- 40/40/20
- Unlimited Protein & Vegetables

This recipe counts as a free food for all plans.

TZATZIKI

1 large cucumber, peeled and seeded and finely
      chopped or grated
1 cup nonfat sour cream
2 cloves garlic, minced
juice of ½ to 1 lemon
fresh dill to taste, finely chopped
salt and pepper

Place cucumber in a colander, add 1 teaspoon salt and toss
well. Leave to drain for 1 hour, then rinse off salt and
squeeze out as much water as possible. I roll it up in a tea
towel and wring. If you like it very thick, you should also
drain the yogurt in a coffee filter so some of the water
drains out. You can do this overnight in the refrigerator.
This should also work with whizzed tofu. Mix everything
together, let stand in refrigerator to blend flavors.

This Recipe Will Work With:

- Super EFA
- 3+2
- Insulin Buster
- Protein Plus One
- 30/50/20
- 50/30/20
- 40/40/20
- Unlimited Protein & Vegetables

This recipe counts as a free food for the above plans.

QUICK BREAKFAST IDEAS

MARKY'S MORNING MOCHA

1 cup strong coffee
the appropriate amount of chocolate-flavored
    whey protein powder
half and half (if you are allowed fat)
2 cups of ice

Place in a blender and frappe until frothy. Pour in a glass.

Other Ideas

- Protein shake with a bagel
- Nonfat cheese quesadilla
- Nonfat cottage cheese and oatmeal
- Protein bar (check label for carbohydrates, fats and proteins)
- Egg Beaters and toast
- Egg-white omelet using smoked turkey breast, bell peppers, mushrooms, onions, or spinach

ABOUT THE AUTHOR

*T*he most sought-after healthcare advice in Los Angeles does not come from an M.D. It comes from a thirty-something dynamo named Tony Perrone. With a Ph.D. in Clinical Nutrition, his working knowledge encompasses East and West, and his specialty is a self-styled combination of western medical doctor, psychiatrist, homeopath, nutritionist, herbalist, energy healer, Chinese medical doctor, and diet guru. His eclectic practice is like consulting many specialties at once, creating an all-encompassing healing regimen for the patient. While he does not practice medicine, he has a thriving practice of making people well.

Although he works with people with every illness imaginable, from AIDS to cancer to high blood pressure, approximately half of his 1,500 patients see him specifically for body-fat reduction. His list of clients reads like a Who's Who of Hollywood, and for this he has been labeled by the media as the "Nutritionist of the Stars." Perrone is responsible for some of the most watched celebrity transformations. His work with Demi Moore and her physical transformation from *The Scarlet Letter* to *Striptease* to *G.I. Jane*, as well as his work with such luminaries as Denzel Washington, Bruce Willis, Angela Bassett, Charlie Sheen, and Paula Abdul, has drawn considerable public attention. Television shows such as *Hard Copy*, *Entertainment Tonight*, and *NBC News* have all profiled Perrone. Mainstream publications such as *W Magazine*, *Women's Wear Daily*, *Los Angeles Magazine*, and *Depeche Mode* (France) have also featured his work.

Perrone has a Ph.D. in Clinical Nutrition, and is a professional member of The American Preventative Medical Association, The American Holistic Health Association, The American Association of Nutritional Consultants, The National Academy of Sports Medicine, The American Council on Exercise, and The International Dance and Exercise Association, and is a Certified Nutritional Consultant (CNC). Perrone is an ex-Navy SEAL trainee, and is the only nutritionist listed in the 1998–1999 American Directory of Who's Who in Executives and Business.

wt. training 3x/wk + 40 min run
   4x/wk 60 min run

②
tuna | crackers | vegetables

chicken | red potato | vegetables
turkey | yam | (exc. corn, peas,
fish | rice | carrots)
ground beef | beans

②
cottage cheese | fruit | non-fat
               | canteloupe | cottage cheese
tuna cup | apple | yams
Breakfast   non fat
─────────   cream cheese
                                     turkey